HEALING
ARTHRITIS

HEALING
ARTHRITIS

Complementary Naturopathic, Orthopedic
& Drug Treatments

PENNY KENDALL-REED, ND
& STEPHEN REED, MD, FRCSC

CCNM
PRESS

Third printing, 2010.

Second edition.

The authors would like to acknowledge the support and encouragement of their parents, throughout their careers and during the writing of this book. We would also like to thank Maria Aulicino, David Schleich, Dr Nick Durand, Dr Aubrey Green, Dr Wayne Potashner, and especially Bob Hilderley for their invaluable contributions to the preparation of this book. For initiating and promoting this book, we would like to thank Jamieson Natural Sources. For more information on Jamieson products, call 1-800-265-5088 or visit their website www.jamiesonvitamins.com

The publisher acknowledges the support of the Government of Canada, Department of Canadian Heritage, Book Publishing Industry Development Program.

ISBN 1-897025-09-2

Edited by Bob Hilderley.
Design by Sari Naworynski.
Back cover photo by José Crespo.

Printed and bound in Canada.

Published by CCNM Press Inc., 1255 Sheppard Avenue East, Toronto, Ontario M2K 1E2 Canada.
ccnmpress@ccnm.edu

BRIEF CONTENTS

DESCRIPTIVE CONTENTS

Osteoarthritis

Symptoms – generally over 60 years of age
– most common in weight bearing joints
 (hips and knees)
– usually affects only one or two joints at a time
– pain on movement of the joint
– progressive joint stiffness and loss of motion
– grinding and crunching in affected joint
– intermittent swelling
– does not involve tissues outside the joints

Treatment – weight loss
– ice or heat and other physical modalities
– glucosamine sulfate, chondroitin sulfate, MSM,
 hyaluronic acid, ginger, devil's claw, curcumin
– acupuncture
– yoga
– essential fatty acids
– analgesics and NSAIDs (non–steroidal
 anti–inflammatory drugs)
– injection therapy
– surgery

Arthritis in the Spine

Symptoms – frequent episodes of back pain lasting weeks
– increased pain with activity
– reduced spine mobility even when not painful
– pain radiating to legs, possible numbness or tingling
– leg pain, numbness, or weakness after walking a
 certain distance

Treatment — weight loss
— physiotherapy, conditioning, back education
— glucosamine/chondroitin/MSM/HA complex
— ginger or devil's claw
— calcium and magnesium
— essential fatty acids
— vitamins B–6 and B–12
— arnica homeopathic
— capsicum topical cream
— kava kava, 5–HTP, St. John's wort (see precautions)
— acupuncture
— chiropractic therapy
— lumbar epidural and facet joint injections
— analgesics and NSAIDs
— surgery

Rheumatoid Arthritis

Symptoms — most common between 30 and 60 years of age
— most commonly affects hands and feet
— commonly affects multiple joints
— affects tissues outside the joints
— joint swelling is prominent
— morning stiffness

Treatment — dietary modifications
— splinting
— ice, heat, and other physical modalities
— massage therapy
— glucosamine sulfate, chondroitin sulfate
— devil's claw
— boswellia
— essential fatty acids
— yoga/massage
— NSAIDs
— DMARDs (disease modifying anti–rheumatic drugs)

– antibiotic therapy
– specific immune modifying drugs (e.g., infliximab)
– surgery

Ankylosing Spondylitis (AS)

Symptoms
– onset of back pain before 40 years old
– low back pain lasting at least 3 months
– back pain relieved by exercise
– pain felt in low back and buttocks
– marked morning stiffness
– can affect hips, shoulders
– can affect eyes, lungs, kidneys

Treatment
– education, physiotherapy, and occupational therapy
– acupuncture and massage
– hydrotherapy
– glucosamine, chondroitin, MSM, ginger, and curcumin
– NSAIDs
– surgery
– radiotherapy

Psoriatic Arthritis

Symptoms
– develops in about 10% of people with psoriasis
– redness and swelling in end finger joints
– can affect a number of joints at one time
– back and pelvis pain
– foot and heel pain

Treatment
– high dose essential fatty acids
– quercitin (natural anti–histamine) for skin lesions
– zinc for skin repair
– glucosamine, chondroitin, MSM, hyaluronic acid,
    and ginger
– remove or reduce animal products from the diet
– anti–inflammatory medications

– topical skin therapy

– DMARDs if severe

Systemic Lupus Erythematosus (SLE)

Symptoms – 90% experience arthralgia or arthritis

– arthritis rarely results in damage or disability

– general symptoms include fever, fatigue, depression, face rash with photosensitivity

– can involve heart, lungs, kidney, and nervous system

Treatment – analgesics

– sunscreen

– zinc and vitamins A, E, and essential fatty acids for the skin

– anti–inflammatory medication

– cortisone

– DMARDs

Crystal Arthritis (Gout)

Symptoms – acute hot, red, painful swelling most commonly of great toe joint

– fever

– associated with high blood levels of uric acid

– common in men in 50th decade

– recent ingestion of red wine, red meat, or seafood

Treatment – rest, splinting, ice

– painkillers plus anti-inflammatory medicine

– ginger, devil's claw, curcumin, bromelain acutely

– injection therapy

– globe artichoke, homeopathic colchicine, cranberry for future prevention

– avoidance of aggravating foods

– allopurinol, colchicine medication

Reactive Arthritis

Symptoms
– acute painful swelling of one joint
– generally younger individuals (18–30)
– history of recent infection
– associated foot and heel pain

Treatment
– rest, splinting, ice
– rule out septic arthritis, gout, etc.
– ginger, devil's claw, curcumin, bromelain
– NSAIDs
– methotrexate, azathioprine
– antibiotic therapy

Septic Arthritis

Symptoms
– acute, hot, red, very painful swelling of one joint
– fever, chills, malaise
– history of recent infection or surgical procedure

Treatment
– rest, splinting, ice
– test joint fluid and blood to determine infectious
  organism
– surgical drainage of joint
– antibiotic therapy
– acidophilus supplement
– glucosamine, chondroitin, MSM, hyaluronic acid

INTRODUCTION

Arthritis is rarely life-threatening, but it is *lifestyle*-threatening. Advances in all fields of medicine have resulted not only in an older population, but an older population of healthy, active people. No longer are those in middle age happy to slow down their pace and give in to aches and pains. Gone are the days when retirement meant settling into the sofa to watch the golden years drift by. Today, individuals of all ages want to play sports, dance, travel, and stay active. There's often just one thing slowing them down – their sore joints!

The population is getting older. The over 55 year-olds made up 21% of the U.S. population in 2001. That will be over 25% in 2010. And these older individuals are staying healthy. Genetically, humans have the potential to live to 120, but disease has always intervened. As we conquer more and more disease, our lifestyle will be dictated by the ability of our bodies to move and function – and by an increasing dependence on our joints.

Arthritis accounts for more impairment of function among middle-aged and older adults than any other disease category. Twice as many people are limited in their mobility by arthritis than by heart disease. Arthritis is the leading cause of physician visits over age 65. The self-reported prevalence of arthritis is 25% in the 45-65 age group and 50% in the over 65 age group. For individuals over 63, at least 10% have knee arthritis significant enough to cause pain and disability; the figure is 5% for hip arthritis. But arthritis is not a disease confined to the middle-aged or the elderly. Arthritis causes debility and pain that can have a significant impact on our enjoyment of life at any age.

It has been shown repeatedly that when individuals understand their illness and take an active part in the treatment, they get a better outcome. This book aims to both educate you about arthritis and inform you of the many treatment options. While, as yet, there is no cure for arthritis, there are many therapies that reduce the symptoms, improve function, and, in some cases, slow progression. With this information, you can make informed choices and, with the help of your health care practitioner, plan a course of action to get you back in motion!

The tenet of this book is *complementary* medicine, the symbiosis of naturopathic and allopathic treatments to achieve a better outcome than either alone. By 'naturopathic' treatments, we mean the medical practice of using natural substances and therapies, such as diet, natural supplements, herbs, homeopathic remedies, acupuncture, and lifestyle changes, to stimulate the body's innate healing response and thus to produce a therapeutic effect. Prevention of disease is a central concept within naturopathic medicine, which emphasizes patient education to reduce the incidence of disease and education of the physical body itself, strengthening its component parts to improve overall health and resist disease.

Naturopathic medicine borrows from many ancient healing traditions, with naturopathic physicians being trained in the use of clinical nutrition, botanical or herbal medicine, homeopathic medicine, traditional Chinese medicine and acupuncture, hands-on techniques, and lifestyle counseling. Training for naturopathic medicine is extensive. A three-year degree of pre-med study at university is followed by a four-year, full-time program at a naturopathic college. In all licensed provinces or states, a naturopathic physician must also pass licensing exams (such as NPLEX in some states and provinces in North America) before being allowed to practice.

By 'allopathic' treatments, we mean traditional pharmaceutical and surgical treatments. Specialists in the field of arthritis include rheumatologists and orthopedic surgeons. Rheumatology is a subspecialty of internal medicine, comprised of the study and treatment of arthritis and many diverse rheumatologic disorders affecting joints and numerous other tissues and organs throughout the body. Orthopedic surgery is the surgical specialty concerned with the locomotor system – the bones, joints, muscles, ligaments, and tendons of the body that provide support and allow movement. From the neck to the feet, orthopedic surgeons treat strains, fractures, dislocations, instabilities, and arthritis. Although we do perform surgeries, including joint replacement, arthroscopy, and fracture repair, we evaluate and coordinate many non-surgical therapies beneficial to the healing and repair of the musculo-skeletal system. After medical school and internship, orthopedic surgeons generally train for 4 years in a residency program before spending 1 to 2 years in subspecialty fellowships, honing their skills in a particular field, such as total joint replacement.

Depending upon the type and severity of arthritis and the nature of the individual, treatment will sometimes be mostly naturopathic, in other cases, mostly allopathic. At one end of the medical spectrum, traditional allopathic medicine can play the predominant role in treatment. We can capitalize on the stronger medications and surgical techniques of traditional medicine, while strengthening the body and preventing further damage though the use of naturopathic medicine. At the other end of the spectrum, naturopathic medicine can take the forefront in treatment by providing adequate relief of symptoms with natural supplementation, repairing previous damage and preventing further destruction, with the option of progressing to traditional medical treatment if needed. Between the two lies a wide spectrum of combination therapies. Each type of healing has its own limitations; however, we feel that by combining them, the overall limitations of treatment are reduced, greatly increasing the potential benefit to the patient. In the opinions of our patients, the best form of medicine is one that combines both forms of therapy. By combining these two forms of medicine, it is possible to get the best therapeutic outcome with the fewest side effects

By utilizing all the information and medical data of naturopathic and allopathic treatments, patients have a wider choice of treatment and are better able to become involved in their own care. In this way, they can learn lifestyle changes that will not only help their arthritis, but their overall health.

Whatever decisions you make when considering either natural or traditional treatments of arthritis, it is important that you consider all other pre-existing health conditions you may have and any other medications you may be taking to ensure that your chosen form of treatment will not interact adversely with any of these. Always consult a health care practitioner when starting a new product. Anything that can heal, can harm, and just because a product comes from a natural source does not mean that it is completely free of adverse effects in all individuals.

Our belief in this complementary philosophy and our experience in treating patients with both forms of medicine has prompted us to write this book. *Healing Arthritis* is the first book to provide comprehensive coverage and explanation of naturopathic and allopathic treatments for arthritis. If the language of arthritis is new to you, you may want to review the 'glossary' at the back of the book to become familiar with basic terminology.

Case Studies

The following case studies show how these complementary forms of treatment can be used to treat patients suffering from various kinds of arthritis, defined at length later in this book.

Osteoarthritis

Dianne is a 58-year-old female with moderate osteoarthritis in her knees. She had been using traditional anti-inflammatories for 2 1/2 years to control her pain. Despite fairly good pain relief, her range of motion, joint stiffness, and activity limitation had continued to deteriorate. Dianne was seeking other means of slowing down the arthritic process as well as relieving her symptoms. As she was approximately 40 pounds overweight, we discussed the increased stress this placed on her joints, and followed up with a weight loss program designed for her.

In addition, Dianne began taking a nutritional supplement combining glucosamine sulfate, chondroitin sulfate, MSM, and hyaluronic acid, together with essential fatty acids. Within 6 weeks she noticed reduced stiffness, improved mobility, and further reduction in pain. Her activity level and her sleep greatly improved. At this point, Dianne began to decrease her dose of traditional anti-inflammatories. Within 2 1/2 weeks she was able to stop them completely. Dianne continues to use the traditional anti-inflammatory medicine on an intermittent basis when her symptoms flare up. However, avoidance of long-term continuous use has made her feel better and reduced her likelihood of developing stomach ulceration.

With improvement in pain and reduced weight, Dianne was able to increase her activity level. A course of physiotherapy helped improve range of motion and strength as well as educating her on the best forms of exercise for her knees.

Rheumatoid Arthritis

Linda is a 52-year-old female with rheumatoid arthritis, predominantly affecting her hands. She developed large, stiff, and swollen joints with little movement or strength. She was already taking glucosamine sulphate and boswellia, and following consultation with a rheumatologist, Linda was started on the drugs prednisone and methotrexate. With this regimen, her pain diminished greatly. She was very pleased with the results and wanted to continue on these medications. However, she was concerned about possible long-term side effects and was interested in preventing them.

Prednisone is known to cause water retention, weight gain, an increase in blood pressure, and cholesterol. To help combat these side effects, Linda followed a naturopathic diet. By reducing her insulin levels through this diet, her kidneys released excess fluid, thereby decreasing the bloating and blood pressure side effects. In addition, by stabilizing insulin levels, she was able to lose some weight (reducing stress on other joints) and then maintain a healthy diet and weight. The naturopathic diet also resulted in decreased cholesterol.

Prednisone also results in loss of bone density, increasing the risk of osteoporosis. To address this side effect, we prescribed calcium, magnesium, zinc, vitamin D, and hydroxyapatite. Together, these supplements provide the building materials for bone and help stimulate bone production.

Methotrexate inhibits folate metabolism. It can irritate the gastrointestinal tract, leading to ulcers, and with prolonged intake, methotrexate also causes liver damage. To help prevent these symptoms and side effects, folic acid supplementation was given along with slippery elm, marshmallow, and cabbage (in herbal form not food) with zinc. Together these act as natural anti-inflammatories and heal the gastro-intestinal tract, treating and preventing lesions. Milk thistle was used to protect and repair the liver, and an increase in water intake was recommended to keep flushing the body.

Psoriatic Arthritis

Sam is a 48-year-old male with psoriatic arthritis. He presented with skin rash over his knees and elbows, along with back and hip pain, heel spurs, and achilles tendonitis.

Sam was taking traditional anti-inflammatories twice a day for the joint pain and was using topical cortisone cream for the skin. However, the cortisone was thinning his skin after prolonged use and the medications were irritating his stomach.

Sam was taking 1 or 2 glucosamine pills twice a day but did not feel they were helping. We decided to start him on glucosamine sulfate, MSM, and ginger for the joint pain. A high dose of essential fatty acids were used for both the skin and the joints. Finally, quercitin, a natural anti-histamine, was used to help with the itchiness and inflammation in the skin.

Sam improved about 65%, greatly reducing his anti-inflammatory use. At this point, we decided to implement dietary changes. Although Sam was not overweight, he consumed a high proportion of animal products. Within 3 weeks of removing all animal products, his symptoms improved once again. Each time he tries to introduce the animal products, he gets a slight flare up, but not nearly as intense as before. Sam was particularly sensitive to diet changes. Whereas some people can re-introduce animal products in small amounts without any ramifications, Sam could not. He then learned that on occasion, when he did want to eat animal products, he could take a traditional anti-inflammatory to mitigate the effect. This was infrequent, markedly reducing the gastric side effects with these medications.

Treatment for his feet and ankles included regular icing, orthotics, a stretching and splinting program, and an injection of cortisone into the more severe of the two heel spurs.

Gout

Rick is a 52-year-old male who over indulges in alcohol and red meat. He presented with gout in his left great toe, causing severe pain and swelling.

Initial treatment to resolve the acute episode included splinting, ice, and indomethacin, a strong anti-inflammatory. To reduce the gastric effects of the indomethacin, zinc, slippery elm, and marshmallow were prescribed.

Once the acute attack was over, Rick sought out natural treatment to help him with his condition. Rick reluctantly eliminated all foods that increased uric acid production in the body, including all shell fish, red meats, old cheese, and dark alcohols, such as red wine and bourbon. In addition, Rick started globe artichoke, milk thistle, cranberry, and colchicine supplements. Within 4 weeks his symptoms were completely cleared. He had no side effects and has had no recurrences.

Osteoarthritis

Doris, a 65-year-old woman, presented with severe osteoarthritis in her left hip. This had been present for many years but had become gradually worse over the past year or so and was now impacting significantly on her life. She could no longer walk her dog or do her gardening, and the limp was causing back pain.

Doris had tried numerous treatments, all of which had helped initially. These included glucosamine sulphate, essential fatty acids, ginger, and devil's claw, along with changes to her diet. She had been unable to tolerate prescription anti-inflammatory medicines due to stomach upset An injection of hyaluronan into the hip had given relief for only 6 weeks.

Following evaluation and x-rays, it was felt that her best option was a total hip replacement. Doris had a good friend who had recently had the same surgery and was already tending to her shrubs!

Prior to surgery, supplements that might adversely affect the procedure were stopped, including essential fatty acids and willow. Protein intake was increased to help with healing after surgery, along with zinc and glucosamine sulphate. Homeopathic arnica was started to reduce inflammation and pain.

Doris underwent a successful hip replacement. Her recovery was rapid and uncomplicated. While she did feel pain from the surgery for the first few days, this was alleviated by the nerve block placed by the anaesthetist and a self-controlled pain-relief pump. Her deep arthritis pain was gone immediately and she was able to start walking within the first few days. Arnica was continued for 1 week. She continues to take a glucosamine/chondroitin/MSM complex preventatively but is pleased she had her surgery. Her dog has never been happier and her garden is a picture!

(1) | WHAT IS ARTHRITIS?

The word *arthritis* literally means inflammation of a joint. Arthritis, however, is perhaps best considered as a *symptom*. It describes an inflamed, stiff, swollen joint, which is the end result of a number of disease processes. While inflammation may be the principal underlying process that has resulted in the symptoms of pain and swelling, its cause may be quite varied. In addition, the disease causing the arthritis may affect other tissues in close proximity, or in some cases at some distance from the joint.

By attaching other descriptions to the word "arthritis" – for example, osteoarthritis or rheumatoid arthritis – we can more closely identify and distinguish the different disease processes and patterns. However, the classification of arthritis has become increasingly difficult in recent years as research into the immunology and biochemistry of arthritis has revealed similarities between conditions previously considered separate entities. The classic division between non-inflammatory or *osteoarthritis* and inflammatory (typically *rheumatoid*) arthritis has become particularly blurred as more and more inflammatory chemicals, such as interleukin-1 (IL-1) and tumor necrosis factor (TNF), are discovered as playing an important part in the development and progression of all forms of arthritis.

No longer does it appear that osteoarthritis is purely the result of wear and tear, or that rheumatoid arthritis is purely the result of immunological over-activity.

The classification of different types of arthritis nevertheless does help to distinguish different patterns of disease by contrasting the presentation of symptoms, clinical findings, and the results of x-rays and blood tests. Such classification is helpful in organizing thought processes as well as in creating guidelines for prognosis and treatment. Unfortunately, not everyone can be slotted conveniently into a particular category or diagnostic group. This emphasizes the importance of individualized patient care and the role of the health care practitioner in establishing a suitable treatment regime.

Anatomy of Arthritis

Arthritis most commonly occurs at a synovial joint. Most of our joints are synovial, including all the major joints, such as the hip, knee, and shoulder. There are several key features of a synovial joint:

- They occur between two bones.
- There is a space or potential space between the bones.
- The bone ends are covered by articular cartilage
    (smooth lubricated cartilage).
- The joint is enclosed in a fibrous capsule.
- The capsule is lined with synovial membrane that produces
    synovial fluid for lubrication of the joint.

Most synovial joints allow significant motion across them, and *all* synovial joints allow at least some motion. The joints are moved by the muscles that cross the joint and are stabilized by the ligaments that surround them. They are designed to be highly congruous – that is, the surfaces conform very closely to each other to allow smooth motion. This becomes very relevant when we talk about the development of arthritis after joint injury or in abnormally formed joints. Articular cartilage is the specialized name given to the tissue or gristle that covers the end of a bone at the joint. This highly organized structure is designed to allow unhindered smooth motion and resist the numerous stressors that occur within a joint.

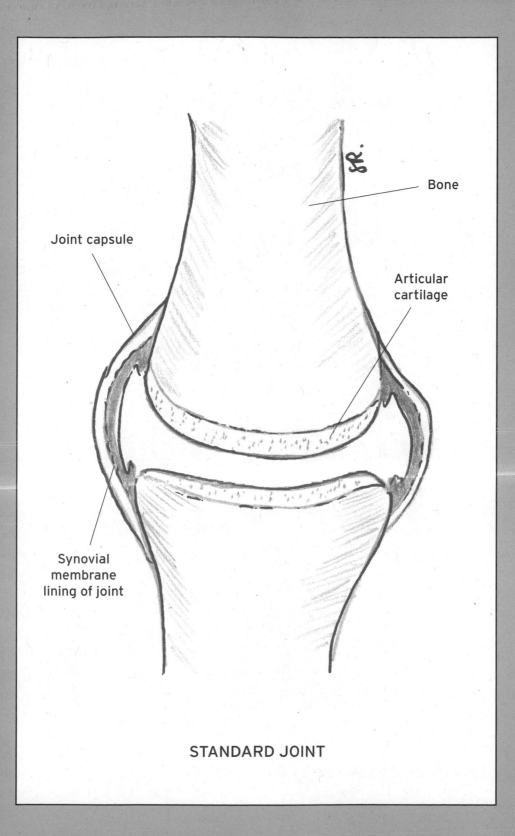

Bone

Joint capsule

Articular
cartilage

Synovial
membrane
lining of joint

STANDARD JOINT

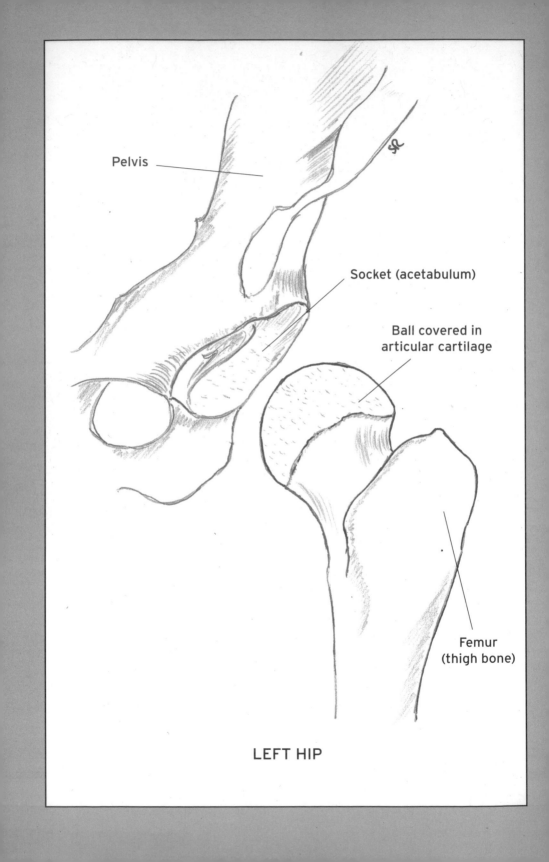

Pelvis

Socket (acetabulum)

Ball covered in
articular cartilage

Femur
(thigh bone)

LEFT HIP

Specific Joints

Hip

The hip is a ball and socket joint between the upper end of the femur or thighbone and the pelvis. A large weight-bearing joint, the hip is very stable and accommodates tremendous forces. For example, during the standing phase of walking or even during raising of a straight leg while lying, the forces across the hip are at least 3 times body weight. In other activities, values as high as 6 times body weight have been calculated. The hip joint is commonly involved in arthritis of all types, second only to the knee in incidence and severity requiring surgical intervention.

Arthritis in the hip generally presents with pain. It is a deep joint so swelling is not usually a primary problem. The pain from hip arthritis is generally felt in the region of the groin but can radiate down into the thigh as far as the knee. It is not uncommon for a patient to be referred to us for assessment of knee arthritis only to find that the patient has severe arthritis in the hip, which is responsible for the knee pain. Hip pain can also radiate up into the back, although this may primarily be due to an altered gait pattern and muscle spasm. It is always important to rule out pathology in the back being responsible for hip pain, although normally this is quite easy to establish on simple questioning and clinical examination. Development of a limp is another common feature of arthritis at the hip, caused by favoring the opposite limb due to pain on the affected side, and by weakness in the muscles that hold the body level when standing on one leg. This so-called 'Trendelenburg sign' makes it difficult to stand on the affected hip without throwing the body weight directly above it so as to minimize forces across the joint.

Stiffness in the hip resulting from osteoarthritis presents with difficulty in common movements, such as cutting toenails or putting on shoes and socks. Stiffness may also result in the inability to straighten the hip fully, resulting in increased arching of the back and subsequent back pain. As the arthritis progresses and movement across the hip joint is lost, the leg may become noticeably shorter. It may also begin to turn outwards, which also affects walking patterns.

Knee

The knee is a complex joint between the lower end of the thighbone or femur and the upper end of the shinbone or tibia. It also incorporates an articulation between the undersurface of the kneecap or patella and the front of the end of the thighbone. The joint is surrounded by a large cavity where fluid accumulations are easily seen. The joint can be considered to have three separate compartments: medial, lateral, and patellofemoral. Arthritis can develop in one or all of these compartments. Osteoarthritis tends to affect the patellofemoral and medial compartments, while rheumatoid arthritis leads to a more generalized deterioration occasionally, with emphasis on the lateral side. The knee, like the hip, is a weight-bearing joint, and during activity such as climbing stairs, similar forces to those encountered in the hip are generated. Three to 6 times body weight can be transmitted across the medial, lateral, or patellofemoral compartments. An important feature of the knee joint is that, unlike the hip, it is not inherently very stable. Stability requires the integrity of the ligaments and the shock absorbing meniscal cartilages. Damage to these early in life can predispose one to the early development of post-traumatic osteoarthritis.

Pain from arthritis in the knee can be sharp and localized as often occurs with degeneration in the medial compartment. There may be a sharp burning pain associated with walking, stair climbing, or direct pressure. This pain may spread down into the medial side of the shin. Similarly, pain from arthritis in the patellofemoral joint is often felt behind the kneecap and is made worse by squatting or climbing stairs. In addition to these sharp localized pains, arthritis in the knee can present with a dull aching or burning felt behind the knee. This pain may spread up into the thigh or down into the calf. The pain is almost always aggravated by activity, and as it becomes more severe, can cause an individual to limp.

Swelling in the knee is quite recognizable due to it being a superficial joint and having a large synovial cavity. Swelling within the knee joint associated with arthritis is generally noted above the kneecap and to either side, filling the two hollows that normally exist there. This should not be confused with bursitis, which usually gives rise to swelling under the skin in the front of the kneecap or just below (as in 'housemaid's knee'). Occasionally, fluid may accumulate in the back of the knee forming a

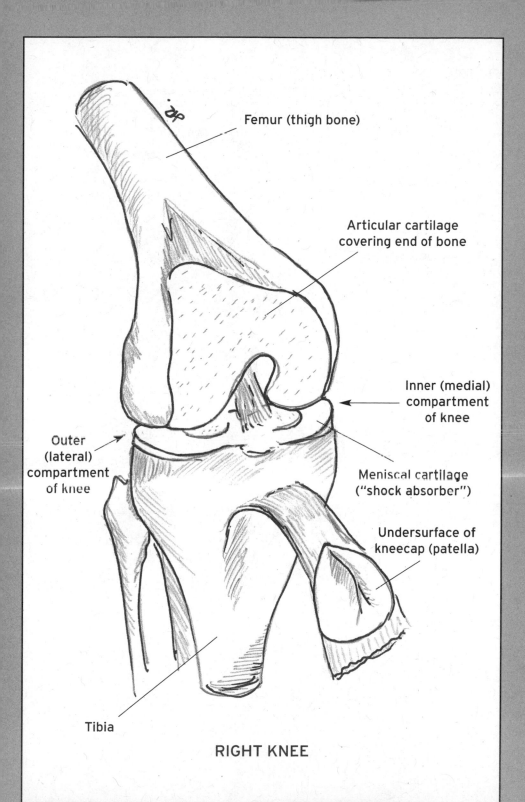

Femur (thigh bone)

Articular cartilage
covering end of bone

Inner (medial)
compartment
of knee

Meniscal cartilage
("shock absorber")

Undersurface of
kneecap (patella)

Outer
(lateral)
compartment
of knee

Tibia

RIGHT KNEE

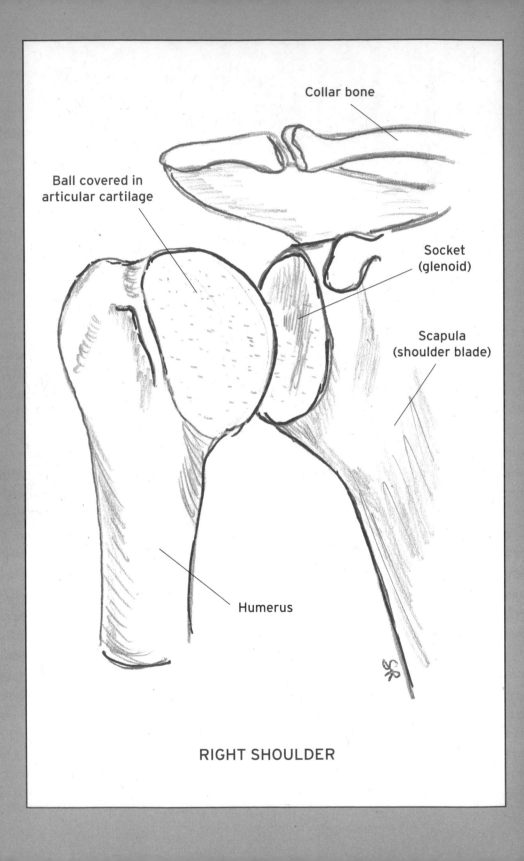

Collar bone

Ball covered in
articular cartilage

Socket
(glenoid)

Scapula
(shoulder blade)

Humerus

RIGHT SHOULDER

so-called Baker's cyst (after the man not the profession). The existence of a Baker's cyst is usually indicative that there is damage causing inflammation inside the knee joint and is particularly associated with arthritis.

In the medial and lateral compartments, acting as a cushion or shock absorber between the end of the femur and the upper surface of the tibia, are the meniscii or meniscal cartilages. These are generally what are referred to in athletes when they "tear a cartilage." These structures are important in cushioning and stabilizing the joint. They improve its congruity and help spread synovial fluid. The meniscii or meniscal cartilages are prone to tearing in younger athletes who present with symptoms of localized sharp joint pain along the inner or outer part of the knee with associated locking, catching, swelling, or giving way. Treatment often involves arthroscopic surgery to repair or trim them. Their importance is gauged by long-term studies of patients who had the entire meniscus removed in the early days of orthopedic surgery. Follow-up studies showed that they rapidly developed arthritis in the compartment were the meniscus was resected. More recent studies show that partial resection is not as disruptive.

As we age, these menisci lose their resilience and flexibility, effectively drying out like a rubber washer. They can crack and split, giving rise to what is called a degenerative tear. These can often cause sharp localized pain along the medial or lateral side of the knee in addition to pre-existing pain from arthritis.

Arthritis in the knee often involves increasing stiffness, including the inability to straighten the knee fully or to achieve a level of flexion whereby an individual can kneel or squat. Arthritis in the knee may present with increasing deformity, such as progressive bowing of the legs or increasing knocked knees. Catching, grinding, and clicking are often found in arthritis of the knees, though not all cracking or clicking is due to arthritis, particularly in young individuals.

Shoulder

The shoulder is a non-weight bearing joint between the ball-like upper end of the arm bone or humerus and a shallow socket formed at the outer edge of the scapular or shoulder blade. Osteoarthritis is uncommon at this joint, it being far more frequently affected by rheumatoid arthritis.

Arthritis may be post-traumatic or related to extensive tearing of the rotator cuff muscles.

Perhaps due to the fact that the shoulder is a non-weight bearing joint and the fact that it normally has extensive mobility, the most common presentation is stiffness. For example, individuals may have difficulty reaching behind the back to do up a brassiere or reaching above the head to wash their hair. Pain in the shoulder is often deep seated. It may be felt as a deep burning or aching in the front of the shoulder. There may be associated pain felt on the outer edge of the shoulder and occasionally pain spreading down into the upper arm through the biceps muscle and sometimes down into the fingers. The pain is often felt in the region of the shoulder blade or the side of the neck as muscles here are often tight and fatigued due to splinting of the joint to protect it against movement and pain. Swelling in the shoulder is uncommon, though it may be excessive in a thin individual.

Arthritis pain in the shoulder usually starts at the shoulder and spreads down into the arm and up into the neck. This can be differentiated from arthritis or other problems in the neck, which generally spread from the neck through the top part of the shoulder as far as the tip of the shoulder and not beyond.

Elbow

The elbow is rarely involved in primary osteoarthritis, although it is a common site for involvement in rheumatoid or inflammatory arthritis. Arthritis in the elbow can develop secondary to trauma, following a serious fracture, for example, or following repetitive trauma, such as occurs in certain occupations. The most common presentation is of loss of range of motion. Generally, there will be an inability to straighten the elbow fully, which may become gradually worse over time. There may also be an inability to bend it fully, which tends to be more disabling with respect to function. There may be associated catching or locking of the elbow. In rheumatoid arthritis, there may be marked associated swelling.

Wrist

Primary osteoarthritis rarely affects the wrist. As with the elbow, the wrist is more commonly affected in post-traumatic arthritis resulting from serious fracture, dislocation, or avascular necrosis. It is more commonly involved as a primary joint in rheumatoid arthritis, where there is marked associated swelling, reduced movement, and deformity. There is generally pain, which is well localized to the region of the wrist joint and associated stiffness.

Thumb

The basal joint of the thumb (carpometacarpal joint) is a site commonly affected by osteoarthritis, particularly in women. There is often associated swelling and deformity of the joint with reduced movement. There is well-localized pain, which is aggravated by pinching and gripping, and if it affects the dominant hand, it can be quite disabling with respect to activities of daily living.

Fingers

The knuckle joints are most commonly affected by inflammatory arthritis, such as rheumatoid arthritis. The joints further down the fingers are more commonly involved in osteoarthritis, where they may show stiffness, deformity, and bony nodules adjacent to the joint. However, arthritis of these joints is not usually painful and rarely requires surgery. Severe involvement of the knuckle joint by rheumatoid arthritis can lead to swelling, deformity, disruption of function, including rupture of tendons, and may require surgical intervention.

Ankle

Osteoarthritis of the ankle is uncommon. It is most commonly related to previous fracture, though even then, the risk is low unless there is substantial disruption of the joint. The risk of developing arthritis following an undisplaced ankle fracture, or one in which essentially normal alignment is restored by casting or surgical treatment, is less than 5%.

Great Toe

The large joint of the great toe (the common site for a bunion) is the most frequently affected by gout, a type of arthritis caused by crystals. Osteoarthritis can often occur at this joint and may be a result of a repetitive trauma, as may be the case with some athletes. In these individuals, the build up of osteophytes or bone spurs can lead to stiffness and pain, particularly on bending the toe upwards as often occurs during running or walking. This condition is called hallux rigidus and can often be treated simply by excision of the bone spur. Arthritis can be associated with bunions but in general the pain from bunions is due to development of a bursitis caused by the rubbing of shoe wear over the angulated joint and co-existing bony spur.

Spine (Neck and Back)

The entire spine is composed of a number of segments or vertebrae, which, like building blocks, are piled one on top of another. They are joined together at the front by discs made of fibrous tissue and cartilage. They are linked at the back by small joints, which are in fact synovial joints (same type as the knee or hip) called facet joints. The spinal cord runs up the middle of this long structure, sending out nerves which emerge at each level to supply tissues both close to and distant from the spine. For example, the nerve that supplies feeling to the big toe actually leaves the spine to begin its journey at the lower part of the back. The bony vertebrae, the discs, and the facet joints do have a degree of inherent stability, but this is not substantial. The spine relies on extensive support from innumerable ligaments and muscles, which run up and down the spine and neck, surrounding the vertebrae. The neck is the part of the spine comprised of the seven vertebral segments between the chest and the base of the skull.

Osteoarthritis

Osteoarthritis is also known as degenerative joint disease (DJD), osteoarthrosis, hypertrophic arthritis, and non-inflammatory arthritis. It is the most common form of arthritis and likely exists to some degree in all individuals by age 65. Over 20 million North Americans over the age of 45 are affected by the disease. Women are affected more than men. Osteoarthritis is not a new disease. It has been identified in the bones of dinosaurs and in the skeletons of pre-historic man and Egyptian pharaohs. It is seen in almost all vertebrates, including those that live in water.

Osteoarthritis is primarily a disease that affects the smooth articular cartilage that covers the ends of our bones within the joint. Articular cartilage is a highly specialized composite of cells, fibers, and matrix 'glue'. It holds water to provide cushioning, yet has the structural integrity to withstand impact and shear force. Its interaction with the synovial fluid that circulates within the joint results in almost frictionless motion. In osteoarthritis, this structure breaks down, resulting in loss of its ability to provide support, resistance, and unhindered movement. The matrix 'glue' becomes weak and the fibers disorganized, leading to over-hydration and softening. Fissures appear and layers of cartilage are lost. Attempts by the few cells to restore order are futile and hindered by the increased production of enzymes that accelerate destruction (collagenases and metalloproteinases). The damaged proteins that are released induce an immune reaction, further increasing inflammation and breakdown.

Osteoarthritis also affects the bone underlying the cartilage (subchondral bone), causing thickening and rigidity along with minute fractures that may be the cause of some of the pain associated with arthritis. The stiffer bone results in more force being transferred to the cartilage, also accelerating breakdown.

The lining of the joint (synovium) becomes inflamed by irritation from the debris of cartilage destruction and the associated immune inflammatory response. It becomes thickened, painful, and produces excess fluid, causing the joint to swell.

Tissues surrounding the joint, such as the capsule, bursa, ligaments, and tendons, are also affected, with thickening causing stiffness, inflammation causing pain, and fluid causing swelling.

Theories of Osteoarthritis

For many years, osteoarthritis was considered to be *chondrogenic*. This means that the primary cause is the breakdown of the articular cartilage. This can certainly occur, resulting from the inflammatory destruction of cartilage by a number of processes. However, it does not account for the overgrowth and remodeling of bone that is seen in osteoarthritis. While it remains possible that cartilage fibrillation is the first event in the progressive deterioration that leads to osteoarthritis, other events occurring around the joint simultaneously and the discovery of initial changes in the subchondral bone would argue against this theory. Interestingly, major areas of remodeling are in the non-weight bearing areas, whereas the major areas of fibrillation are in the weight bearing areas of the joint, which indicates different causation. It is possible that development of increased stiffness in the subchondral bone leading to micro fracture may precede the cartilage damage. Increased stiffness following repair of these micro fractures results in the overlying cartilage absorbing a greater portion of the transmitted energy during weight bearing.

Osteoarthritis does not appear simply to be the result of wear and tear over time. There appear to be a number of factors that influence its onset, progression, and characteristics. It is likely that osteoarthritis represents a final pathway for a number of different etiologies which, when they occur together, can combine to affect disease development, severity, and progression.

Primary Osteoarthritis

Osteoarthritis has classically been divided into primary osteoarthritis, in which the clearly identified etiological factor is age, and secondary osteoarthritis, in which there is some well defined pre-disposing factor, such as joint damage or abnormality. However, as with differences between inflammatory and non-inflammatory arthritis, the division between primary and secondary osteoarthritis is becoming blurred. It is likely that in the future, specific etiologies will be identified in primary osteoarthritis patients, effectively placing them into the secondary osteoarthritis category.

Although primary osteoarthritis is classically defined as being idiopathic (of unknown origin), recent studies have identified possible etiologies and risk factors which are likely at play in the majority of cases. The presence of inflammatory chemical mediators, such as cytokines, indicate a more complex disease process than a simple rubbing away of cartilage by daily wear and tear.

The following factors have been found related to the development and progression of osteoarthritis:

Obesity

There appears to be a definite link between obesity and the development of osteoarthritis. The association of obesity and occupations that involve prolonged kneeling and squatting has been implicated in the development of osteoarthritis of the knees. Weight loss in established osteoarthritis can certainly result in significant improvement in symptoms. This in part may be simply due to biomechanical factors, but there may be an important role in promotion of healing and avoidance of further deterioration. Dietary and hormonal abnormalities associated with obesity may also have an important role in the etiology of osteoarthritis.

Exercise and Activity
There is increasing evidence that excessive weight bearing activity in athletes or in certain occupations may be an important etiology in the development of osteoarthritis. While there is no evidence that low-level recreational competitive activity leads to osteoarthritis, excessive participation in high impact sports over a long period of time at an elite level can be associated with osteoarthritis, even in the absence of significant trauma. There is an increased association between arthritis of the hip and knee joints in soccer, rugby, racket sports, and track and field. All these, however, are associated with performance at a high level.

Biomechanics
Biomechanics refers to the overall shape, alignment, and balance of the joint. The presence of abnormal biomechanical alignment, such as excessive bowing of the legs, excessive knock-knee alignment, and abnormal tracking of the kneecap, is not only associated with increased risk of overuse injury but also with the development of osteoarthritis. This is particularly so in cases where there are numerous factors at play, such as biomechanical abnormality, obesity, and excessive loading of the joint.

Hormonal Influence
There is clear evidence that the age period coinciding with the peak of menopause is associated with the increased development of osteoarthritis. The increased incidence of osteoarthritis in women, and the influence of estrogenic hormones in the development, symptoms, and progression of the disease, all point to a hormonal role for estrogen. So far, no association between menstrual or obstetric history has been established. Estrodiol (a synthetic estrogen) worsens experimental arthritis, and disease symptoms are relieved by tamoxifen (an estrogen blocker). Insulin like growth factor

(IGF-1) may play a role in the development of osteoarthritis. Studies have indicated a disruption in the normal relationship between IGF-1 and bone and cartilage metabolism. It is possible that changes induced in the subchondral bone by local activation of IGF-1 may well be initiating factors in the development of cartilage breakdown of osteoarthritis.

Nerve Supply

There is increasing evidence for the role of altered joint sensation in the development of osteoarthritis. In the extreme case of a neuropathic or 'Charcot' joint, which occurs following nerve dysfunction in diabetes, for example, the loss of sensory feedback results in massive destruction of the joint and surrounding tissue. There is evidence that the loss of sensory feedback resulting from torn ligaments may be partially responsible for the development of early arthritic change following trauma.

Genetic Predisposition

Some studies have indicated a definite predisposition to osteoarthritis. It is likely, however, that this is related mainly to a genetic predisposition to other etiological factors, particularly biomechanics and joint dysplasia (abnormal joint formation).

Secondary Osteoarthritis

It is likely that this category of arthritis only exists because one of the many etiological factors in a multi-factorial disease is prevalent and clearly related to the development of the condition. It is likely, however, that all forms of osteoarthritis involve a number of factors, including trauma to the joint.

Fracture

Disruption of the joint surface resulting from trauma, such as occurs in a fracture, is clearly associated with the development of osteoarthritis. In this case, it is commonly called post-traumatic osteoarthritis. The risk for development of post-traumatic osteoarthritis is directly related to the degree of damage that occurred at the time of the fracture. Although accurate surgical reconstruction of the joint surface in cases of severe trauma will improve overall outcome, in general the development of osteoarthritis relates directly to the severity of the trauma.

Bone Bruising

A recent injury identified at the joint surface is that of a bone bruise. The injury was only made visible by the availability of MRI examination of the joint following trauma. Classically, it occurs following a significant ligamentous injury to the knee, such as may occur following tearing of the anterior cruciate ligament. Although direct examination of the joint surface may not reveal any damage, MRI shows evidence of fracture and inflammation in the subchondral bone. This would be analogous to a bruise on an apple where the surface appears intact but on cutting through the skin there is a significant brown bruise identified inside. These bone bruises appear to be areas of damage with potential for early breakdown of the overlying articular surface and possibly the development of osteoarthritis.

Infection

Severe infection within a joint may result in damage to the articular cartilage that results in the development of osteoarthritis.

Ligament Injury

Significant ligamentous injury to a joint may lead to the early development of osteoarthritis. This may be due to impaired nervous feedback from the joint, altered biomechanics, and the co-existence of bone bruises noted above. It is recognized particularly in the knee, where ongoing instability due to ligamentous incompetency results in increased joint damage over time. While repair of the ligament with subsequent restoration of joint anatomy and stability may help prevent further trauma, the damage done at the time of the original injury appears to impose a considerable risk factor for the development of early osteoarthritis in the joint.

Joint Dysplasia

Abnormal development of a joint can lead to the development of early osteoarthritis. This is particularly prevalent at the hip were abnormal formation of a normally congruent ball and socket joint leads to altered articulation and biomechanics. It is possible that there is a wide spectrum of dysplasia, much of which is beyond our ability to detect. In this case, there is clearly overlap with the biomechanical risk factors noted above.

Surgery

Certain surgical treatments can be associated with an increase risk of osteoarthritis. In the days before arthroscopy of joints, a large incision was commonly made to treat such minor pathology as a small meniscus (shock absorbing cartilage) tear. Complete removal of the meniscus was encouraged, but it is now known that this is associated with the early development of osteoarthritis. More recent studies have shown that limited resection through arthroscopic techniques is much less likely to progress towards degenerative change.

Surgery at one joint may adversely affect the biomechanics at another. This is particularly the case with respect to arthrodesis or fusion of the joint, such that no movement is allowed following the surgery. This transfers increased forces to the joints above and below. This is most notable with respect to the hip and the knee and also to the spine were surgical immobilization between two levels invariably leads to increased stress and the development of osteoarthritis at the levels above or below.

Avascular Necrosis

This is a condition in which the blood supply to an area of bone is lost, resulting in bone death and collapse. This may be related to trauma following hip dislocation or fracture of the scaphoid bone in the wrist, for example. In other cases, it may be due to other factors and occur in the absence of any significant trauma. The subsequent abnormalities in the bone and overlying cartilage, along with altered biomechanics of the joint, are likely responsible for the development of osteoarthritis in these cases.

Symptoms

Everyone experiences aches and pains with occasionally stiff joints. This is particularly true of active individuals participating in strenuous work or sports. Muscle pain usually comes on after one to two days, so the cause may not be immediately apparent and may require thinking back to events in the last 48 hours. Simple treatment (ice or heat or simple medication), along with a little time, is usually sufficient to allow these pains to settle. If they do not resolve, or indeed get more severe, then it is time to visit your doctor.

There are, however, certain symptoms or complaints that may indicate you have arthritis. Your doctor or orthopedic surgeon will be the one to confirm or allay your suspicions.

The following list represents a quick guide to osteoarthritis symptoms that indicate a need to see a doctor.

Osteoarthritis Symptoms

Urgent
✦ a hot, painful, swollen joint with fever, malaise, general illness
✦ simultaneous involvement of a number of joints with pain and swelling, possibly associated with skin rash and general illness
✦ joint or limb pain associated with loss of feeling, weakness, or loss of bowel or bladder control

Non-Urgent
✦ joint pain persisting for more than a few days and severe enough to interfere with daily life
✦ joint pain associated with swelling (fluid within the joint)
✦ recurrent pain in one or more joints
✦ pain associated with loss of motion
✦ pain with locking of the joint, or a feeling of giving way

Pain

The pain from osteoarthritis is generally a burning ache, aggravated by movement but causing discomfort at rest. It usually comes on quite rapidly (sometimes associated with swelling), and lasts days to weeks before settling down. Over time, there is a step-wise deterioration, such that each episode may last longer and be more severe.

Swelling

Swelling is not always associated with osteoarthritis, although acute flares may be accompanied by increased joint fluid. Swelling is a more prominent feature of inflammatory arthritis, such as rheumatoid arthritis, and tends to be a more prominent symptom than pain, at least in the early stages of the disease. A joint that becomes rapidly swollen, hot, stiff, and painful, without any injury, should be checked urgently by your doctor.

Stiffness

Loss of motion in a joint can occur in the presence of swelling. Loss of motion without swelling that lasts for weeks and gets progressively worse over time, limiting function and activity, is often due to arthritis.

Grinding

Crunching or grinding is not necessarily due to arthritis. Many joints crack or make noise. The more severe the grinding, and its association with pain, swelling, or stiffness, the more likely it is due to arthritis.

Reduced Function

Altered ability to function that gets progressively worse may indicate arthritis. This generally occurs over months or years and may only be noticed by others. A limp, with diminishing tolerance to walk distances or an inability to cut toenails or wash hair, are more obvious changes and accompany more severe arthritis.

Age

Generally, the older you are the more likely your joint symptoms are due to arthritis. Unless you have had major damage to a joint through fracture, ligament damage, surgery, or infection, arthritis is uncommon below age 45-50.

Arthritis of the Neck and Spine

Arthritis affecting the neck and spine is extremely common and increases with age. Most individuals over the age of 45 will show some evidence of wear or deterioration on x-ray. Fortunately, in the majority of cases these changes do not cause any symptoms. In fact, the individual may be completely unaware that they have any arthritis until they inadvertently injure themselves, sustaining a lumbar or cervical strain injury, and have x-rays taken. They are then told that they have arthritis and immediately find themselves labeled with a chronic and debilitating disease. In a condition so bestowed with emotional and psychological factors, this can only serve to impair recovery from injury. Once again, to emphasize, by far the majority of all neck and back pain has nothing to do with arthritis.

Arthritis of the spine affects both the intervertebral disc and the small synovial type facet joints at the back of the spine. Degeneration of the intervertebral discs may result in disc pain. This type of back pain is typically worse on forward bending and is eased by straightening or arching the spine backwards. Disc herniation with subsequent compression of nerve roots can give rise to leg or arm pain with numbness and tingling or weakness of muscles in severe cases.

Arthritis involving the facet joints has been implicated as a factor in certain types of back pain. This pain is described as typically worse with extension of the back rather than forward flexion, and generally results in severe localized back pain with local radiation only.

Spinal stenosis results from a combination of arthritis and degenerative change affecting the intervertebral disc, the facet joints, and the surrounding ligaments. In this condition, the available space for the spinal cord and emerging nerves is compromised. This may result in radiating pain, such as sciatica, with numbness and tingling or weakness, such as might occur with a disc herniation. It may present with backache in the absence of any nerve entrapment. It may also present in what is termed neurogenic claudication. This is a condition in which pain in the back and nerve symptoms in the legs become progressively worse with activity. When this affects the legs, it can often be confused with vascular claudication, which results from insufficient blood supply to the muscles of the legs associated with smoking and artery disease. The main difference is that claudication due to a problem in the spine is not relieved simply by stopping and standing still. It usually requires sitting or bending forward to relieve the pressure on the spine.

Rheumatoid Arthritis

Rheumatoid arthritis is one of a number of inflammatory diseases that diffusely affect tissues throughout the body. These diseases also include psoriatic arthritis, ankylosing spondylitis, Reiter's syndrome, SLE (systemic lupus erythematosus), dermatomyositis, and vasculitis.

The distinguishing feature of rheumatoid arthritis is it predilection for affecting primarily synovial joints. Other diseases in this group can also affect the joints, but the arthritis tends to be a less prominent symptom as other tissues are more frequently involved (for example, the skin in psoriatic arthritis).

The major differences distinguishing osteoarthritis from rheumatoid arthritis are listed in the table below:

	Osteoarthritis	Rheumatoid Arthritis
Age	over 65	Women 30-50 Men 50-70
Common joints affected	knees/hips	hands/feet
Number joints affected	1 or 2, usually 1 side first	multiple joints, both sides
Systemic symptoms (fatigue, fever, etc.)	absent	can occur
Non-joint involvement (lungs, skin, heart, etc.)	absent	common
Blood tests	normal	rheumatoid factor

Rheumatoid arthritis is the most common type of inflammatory arthritis and affects about 1% of the population. Women tend to develop rheumatoid arthritis in their thirties and forties with men developing it in their fifties and sixties. By age 65, it is estimated that approximately 0.75% of women and 0.2% of men suffer from rheumatoid arthritis.

Theories of Rheumatoid Arthritis

Despite many advances in the study of rheumatology over the past few decades, the cause of rheumatoid arthritis remains unknown. As with osteoarthritis, it is likely that there are multiple factors involved. There does appear to be a genetic pre-disposition, and environmental studies have shown an increased incidence in metropolitan as compared to rural areas. There appears to be hormonal influence with remission of disease in the last trimester of pregnancy and a subsequent flare-up of the disease following birth. Infectious agents have been implicated in rheumatoid arthritis, although research has failed to reveal a responsible or transmissible organism. Although the demographics of the disease do not fit an infectious cause, it is possible that an infectious agent plays a role in stimulating the onset or progression of rheumatoid arthritis through a disturbance of the body's immune system, either systemically or localized to the joint.

The concept of rheumatoid arthritis as an auto-immune disease (a condition were the body attacks its own tissues rather than those that are foreign or infectious) was popular for many years. However, this etiology has been questioned. The presence of *rheumatoid factors* (antibodies directed against the body's own immune chemicals or immunoglobulins) has been found to amplify the disease, but these factors do not seem to be its principal cause. A similar finding is made with respect to antibodies directed against collagen, the body's structural tissue.

The main problem in rheumatoid arthritis seems to be the presence and activity of inflammatory cells in numerous tissues, in particular the synovium or lining of the joints. The chemicals produced by these cells promote inflammation and tissue destruction. These products include the interleukins, tumor necrosis factor, leukotrienes, prostaglandins, and metalloproteinases (enzymes shown to break down cartilage).

The destruction of joints associated with rheumatoid arthritis is a combination of two factors. One is direct cartilage damage by the numerous chemicals and enzymes released into the joint. The second is by the uncontrolled growth of the synovium within the joint that is initiated in the rheumatoid process. This pervasive tissue growth invades both the cartilage and the bone surrounding the joint.

Symptoms

Rheumatoid arthritis has a number of different presentations, most of which involve more than one joint, unlike osteoarthritis, where, in the majority of cases, there is a gradual onset of pain in one particular joint. Despite the fact that osteoarthritis may *affect* a number of joints, it is usually one in particular that initially becomes bothersome. Others may develop symptoms later. Rheumatoid arthritis may also present with involvement of one joint, but this is unusual. It most often presents with involvement of a number of joints. Osteoarthritis rarely presents with rapid development of pain unless perhaps there has been an injury to the joint, which was previously not recognized as having arthritis. Trauma to an arthritic joint can often be the straw that breaks the camel's back and initiates symptoms requiring treatment. An individual with classic pain, swelling, and stiffness in hands, wrists, and other joints, along with fatigue, rash, or weight loss is far more likely to be showing early signs of rheumatoid arthritis.

Presentations of Rheumatoid Arthritis

Onset	Rapid (days to weeks)	50%
	Insidious (weeks to months)	50%
Joints involved	Hands and feet	30%
	Elbows, wrists	20%
	Hips, knees	30%
Number of joints	1	20%
	2-3	45%
	>3	35%

The joints most commonly involved with the initial onset of rheumatoid arthritis are the metacarpo-phalangeal joints or knuckle joints of the hands, the first joints of the fingers, and the wrists. This is in contrast to osteoarthritis, where it is generally the major weight bearing joints, such as the hips and the knees, which are first affected. The larger joints are generally affected later in rheumatoid arthritis.

The presentation for rheumatoid arthritis symptoms is extremely varied. It is important to realize that not everyone who develops swelling, pain, and stiffness in a number of joints has rheumatoid arthritis. There are many other causes, including injury or infection, and even cases where no cause can be identified. Over 50% of individuals will show complete resolution over time.

Ankylosing Spondylitis

Ankylosing spondylitis is one of a group of diseases called the spondyloarthropathies. These include ankylosing spondylitis, reactive arthritis, Reiter's syndrome, arthropathy associated with inflammatory bowel disease, and psoriatic arthritis. These diseases are considered a separate entity from rheumatoid arthritis and osteoarthritis, although presentation and involvement of certain joints may be similar.

The incidence of ankylosing spondylitis in the general population is about 0.2%. However, in individuals possessing the genetic marker HLA-B27 the incidence is approximately 1% to 2%.

The etiology or cause of ankylosing spondylitis remains elusive. Strong association with the HLA-B27 genetic marker indicates a possible combination of genetic predisposition and environmental stimulus. Infective agents, such as the Klebsiella organism, have been indicated. There is definite link between another of the spondylo arthropathies, Reiter's syndrome, and the organisms chlamydia, shigella, salmonella, and yersina.

Symptoms

By far the most common presentation of ankylosing spondylitis is low back pain. Low back pain is an extremely common problem affecting a large proportion of the population and not all back pain equals arthritis.

The following symptoms do indicate the possibility of ankylosing spondylitis:

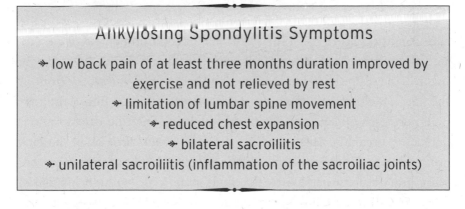

Ankylosing Spondylitis Symptoms

✤ low back pain of at least three months duration improved by exercise and not relieved by rest
✤ limitation of lumbar spine movement
✤ reduced chest expansion
✤ bilateral sacroiliitis
✤ unilateral sacroiliitis (inflammation of the sacroiliac joints)

Five factors differentiate inflammatory back pain induced by spondylitis from back pain of other causes:

– onset of back discomfort before age 40
– insidious onset
– persistence for at least 3 months

– associated with morning stiffness

– improvement with exercise

The back pain is usually felt in the upper buttock and comes on gradually. The pain may move from side to side and is associated with stiffness that is worse in the morning. The pain typically is worse at rest and is eased as the individual begins to mobilize. The pain can spread throughout the back, between the shoulder blades, and occasionally chest pain can be felt either at the back of the chest or in the region of the breastbone.

The hips and shoulders are the most common large joint targets for ankylosing spondylitis and are affected in about 20% of sufferers. In some cases, the pain or stiffness in one of these joints may spark the initial diagnosis.

One feature that ankylosing spondylitis and indeed the other spondyloarthropathies have in common with rheumatoid arthritis and not with osteoarthritis is the involvement of other tissues besides the bones and joints. Ankylosing spondylitis can affect the eyes, heart, lung, and kidneys.

Psoriatic Arthritis

Psoriatic arthritis is a type of inflammatory arthritis associated with the skin condition psoriasis. (Psoriasis is a skin condition characterized by well-demarcated, red lesions covered with silvery scales. It typically involves the scalp and behind the ears, the back of the elbows, the front of the knees, the back, and the buttocks. Involvement of the finger and toenails may resemble a fungal infection with pitting, splitting, discoloration, and debris under the nails). Psoriasis occurs in about 1% to 2% of the general population and psoriatic arthritis develops in about 10% of people with psoriasis. Psoriatic arthritis does not occur without psoriasis, although areas of skin involvement may be minor and may require careful searching for by the physician or patient. Men and women are equally affected with psoriatic arthritis.

Psoriatic arthritis has been identified as distinct from rheumatoid arthritis. The incidence of positive blood test for rheumatoid factor is low. Psoriatic arthritis differs from osteoarthritis in the fact that it is predominately inflammatory and involves tissues other than the joints, most notably the skin and nails. It is different from rheumatoid arthritis in that it tends to involve the joints at the ends of the fingers rather than at the knuckles. It is similar to ankylosing spondylitis in its association with HLA-B27, and is considered one of the spondyloarthropathies.

As with many of the inflammatory arthritides, the exact cause of psoriatic arthritis is unknown. There is certainly a strong genetic component and involvement of the HLA-B27 gene as well as other HLA genes. There is suggestion that there may be a specific psoriasis gene. There is evidence of auto-immunity (where the body's immune system attacks its own tissues), and relationships have been found between viral and bacteria infections and the onset or progression of the disease. There is also indirect evidence that an episode of trauma in a patient with psoriasis may precipitate the development of arthritis.

Symptoms

Psoriatic arthritis can present in five patterns:

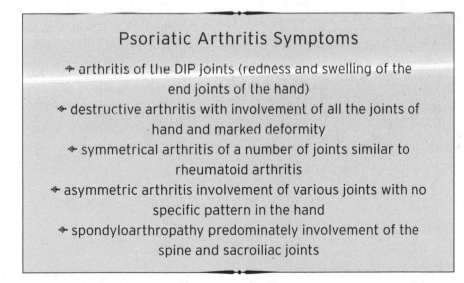

Psoriatic Arthritis Symptoms

✦ arthritis of the DIP joints (redness and swelling of the end joints of the hand)
✦ destructive arthritis with involvement of all the joints of hand and marked deformity
✦ symmetrical arthritis of a number of joints similar to rheumatoid arthritis
✦ asymmetric arthritis involvement of various joints with no specific pattern in the hand
✦ spondyloarthropathy predominately involvement of the spine and sacroiliac joints

Other features included development of foot pain related to plantar fasciitis (heel spurs) and inflammation of the Achilles' tendon or heel cord.

Systemic Lupus Erythematosus (SLE)

SLE is an inflammatory condition affecting numerous tissues throughout the body with over 90% of affected individuals experiencing arthralgia or arthritis. The big difference between arthritis in SLE and rheumatoid arthritis is the lack of cartilage and bone damage. Overall, the arthritis tends to be much milder and more responsive to treatment. It is rare that individuals with SLE will become disabled due to their arthritis or require surgical intervention.

While the specific cause of SLE is unknown, it appears to be a combination of genetic and environmental factors. Of all cases, 90% occur in women with onset between the ages of 15 and 25.

The inflammation and tissue damage in SLE results from an abnormal immune response with production of antibodies against the bodies own tissues. It is suspected that certain individuals have a genetic predisposition to SLE. When exposed to certain environmental factors, including ultraviolet light, sex hormones, dietary factors, and infectious agents, they develop the disease. The characteristic findings in SLE are of antibodies directed against the nucleus DNA of cells (anti-nuclear antibodies or ANA) and anti DNA antibodies. While all individuals produce numerous antibodies that react with the body's own tissue, these antibodies are generally weak and react with many different proteins. In SLE and other auto-immune conditions, the auto antibodies tend to be more aggressive (IgG as opposed to IgM), they seem to have greater infinity for the body's tissues, and they induce a greater inflammatory response. These auto antibodies are the basis of diagnostic tests for SLE.

Symptoms

SLE typically presents with the following symptoms:

SLE Symptoms

✦ fever, loss of appetite and loss of weight
✦ fatigue and depression (85%)
✦ skin changes (butterfly rash on the face, discoid lupus rash)

➤ hair loss (alopecia) and photo-sensitivity (80%)
➤ Raynaud's phenomena (a condition which, on exposure to cold, one or more fingers go white and lose feeling, and on re-warming, there is a burning feeling and intense purple discoloration)
➤ mouth or nose ulceration (30%)
➤ pleurisy or pericarditis (inflammation of the tissue covering the lungs and heart presenting with sharp chest or lung pain worse with deep breathing and coughing)
➤ kidney disease (causes swelling of the tissues and a frothy protein in the urine, but may only be detected with clinical test)
➤ central nervous system and psychiatric conditions (66%), including seizures, psychiatric illness and disorders, and nerve abnormalities in the face

As with the other inflammatory forms of arthritis, in particular rheumatoid arthritis, SLE is a long-term condition that requires careful monitoring and a close association between the individual and the treating physician or rheumatologist. As with rheumatoid arthritis, the presentation, course, and severity of the disease are variable and each individual should be considered as a separate entity.

Crystal Associated Arthritis

In crystal associated arthritis or gout, inflammation of the joint results from irritation by crystals of certain chemicals being deposited directly within the joint. The two main types are *gout,* caused by crystals of uric acid, and *pseudogout,* caused by crystals of calcium pyrophosphate.

Gout

The classic image of an overweight Renaissance nobleman sitting with a bandaged foot elevated on a chair, a glass of port in one hand and a leg of mutton in the other, represents one of the most common presentations of gout. Gout is unique to humans. It is associated with an elevated level of uric acid in the blood.

Symptoms

Acute and painful swelling of the joint at the base of the big toe associated with redness and often fever are common symptoms of gouty arthritis. Acute gouty arthritis usually affects a single joint, most commonly the base of the great toe. Gout can also affect the ankles, knees, wrists, fingers, and elbows. Often the individual wakes with pain and swelling in the affected joint, which rapidly progresses to severe discomfort with associated redness, heat, and swelling. The joint becomes almost impossible to move, making walking difficult, and is very tender to touch. There may be fever or chills.

Gout is associated with raised blood levels of uric acid, a condition that can result in:

– recurrent acute arthritis of joints
– deposits of crystals in the tissues surrounding joints
– kidney stones
– kidney disease and failure

While the incidence of elevated blood uric acid levels is quite high and estimated at between 2% and 20% of the population, few of these individuals, it would seem, develop the symptoms of gout, including arthritis. It usually affects men in their 50th decade. It is associated with obesity, high blood pressure, high cholesterol, hardening of the arteries, diabetes, and conditions in which the kidneys are not functioning efficiently. There is an association with alcohol consumption and the recent ingestion of rich foods, including red meat and cheese. Gout can follow an acute illness, trauma, surgery, or radiation. It is associated with certain blood diseases in which there is destruction of blood cells.

Pseudogout

Pseudogout is an inflammatory arthritis of the joints caused by crystals of calcium pyrophosphate. It is also known as calcium pyrophosphate deposition disease (CPDD) and is associated with the laying down of calcium salts in and around the structural parts of the joints.

The exact cause of CPDD is not known. It primarily affects individuals over 50 years of age and is associated with osteoarthritis. A classic finding is the deposition of calcium in the meniscal cartilage of the knee as seen on x-ray. In chronic pseudogout, the findings are almost identical to osteo-arthritis. Certainly, it is often unclear as to whether the calcium deposits preceded or followed the arthritic changes and destruction of cartilage in the joint.

Acute arthritis associated with pseudogout usually occurs in larger joints, such as the knee and less frequently the wrist and ankle. Unlike gout, the feet and specifically the great toe are rarely affected. Pseudogout may present much like gout or acute infection with sudden pain, swelling, and immobility. The attacks may be brought on by trauma, surgery, or severe medical illness, such as heart attack, much as with regular gout. Occasionally, there are chills and fevers.

Reactive Arthritis

Reactive arthritis refers to the development of an acute inflammatory arthritis involving pain and swelling following an infection. However, the infection does not directly involve the joint, and the site of the infection is often remote from the area of arthritis. The infection usually precedes the arthritis by between 1 and 4 weeks. In many cases, an infectious agent cannot be identified, but a diagnosis is made on the basis of exclusion and certain positive tests.

Symptoms
The presentation of reactive arthritis is quite often acute and maybe confused with infection or gout. This form of arthritis often occurs in a younger patient population.

Reactive Arthritis Symptoms

✦ history of recent infection, including bowel organisms, such as salmonella, urinary tract or sexually acquired organisms, such as chlamydia; fluid drained from the joint contains no organisms but does contain inflammatory cells

✦ tissue inflammation, such as heel spurs, Achilles' tendonitis, and rib inflammation

✦ presence of the HLA- B27 gene product

✦ associated inflammation at remote sites such as the eye and mouth

The majority of patients with reactive arthritis or Reiter's disease show an initial attack lasting 2 to 3 months, followed by prolonged remissions, and 20% to 50% develop a chronic course of peripheral arthritis. This is more common in individuals demonstrating the involvement of joints, eyes, and urinary tract. However, even in those developing chronic inflammation, the disease is not as disabling as rheumatoid arthritis, for example, and amounts to less than 15% percent risk over a lifetime.

Infectious Arthritis

In this form of arthritis, the inflammatory process is a direct result of invasion by bacteria or other organisms and the body's immune reaction against them. The early identification and treatment of infectious arthritis is of utmost importance due to its ability to rapidly cause joint destruction and systemic illness.

Sources

Infection of a joint essentially arises from two possible sources:

1.   from the blood.
2.   from direct inoculation (penetrating injury to the joint, medical treatment, such as injection or surgery, or spread from adjacent structures).

The majority of infections are caused by organisms normally found on the skin, including staphylococcus aureus and epidermidis. Certain other bacteria are frequently released into the blood even in day-to-day activity, such as brushing the teeth. Fortunately, the number or organisms in this situation is extremely small and generally of no consequence. The larger the number of bacteria in the blood, the more likely they are to spread to a joint. The lining of the joint or synovium has an extensive network of blood vessels, which seems to trap certain organisms. The presence of associated conditions, such as rheumatoid or other inflammatory arthritis, recent trauma, or an existing joint replacement, seems to make a joint more susceptible to colonization by circulating bacteria. It is for this reason that individuals with joint replacements and in some cases those with rheumatoid arthritis are encouraged to take antibiotics if they are undergoing any sort of medical procedure that is likely to lead to a marked increase in number of circulating bacteria. This might include dental surgery, surgery on the bowel or urinary system, or in the event that these individuals have an infection, such as a boil or abscess.

Direct inoculation of bacteria into the joint can occur following penetrating trauma. Any significant injury in which the joint is penetrated should be treated with aggressive surgical cleaning. Removal of fluid from a joint through a needle or an injection of anaesthetic, cortisone, or hyaluronate carry a risk of infection and should always be done with appropriate sterile conditions, equipment, and skin cleaning. The risk, however, is extremely low.

Infection following arthroscopic surgery is extremely rare with estimates of between .01 % and .48 %. The risk is increased with prolonged procedure time. The risk of infection following total joint replacement is generally considered to be less than 1%. The risk is slightly higher following revision procedures in which a loose or failed joint replacement is removed and a new one implanted.

Acute Bacterial Arthritis

Acute bacterial arthritis generally presents as an acutely painful and swollen joint. Typically, only one joint is affected. The pain is so severe it may be almost impossible to move the joint. The joint is often hot and red, and there may be inflammation in the tissues and skin surrounding the joint. The individual may feel unwell, with a fever and chills, fatigue, nausea, and vomiting.

Gonococcal Arthritis

Infection caused by neisseria gonorrheae, the organism that causes gonorrhea, can also cause disseminated gonococcal infection (DGI). In contrast to other forms of infectious arthritis, DGI presents with involvement of a number of joints and tendons, as well as a skin rash. Individuals are usually young, healthy, and sexually active. The time frame between sexual contact and the onset of DGI varies from 24 hours to 2 months. Only 25% of individuals have genital or urinary symptoms. A quarter of patients have had a previous history of gonorrhea infection. Treatment involves high dose intravenous or intramuscular antibiotics. The response is usually dramatic. Surgical treatment is not usually required, but removal of fluid from the joint may be required for diagnosis.

Conditions Mistaken for Arthritis

We have lost track of the number of patients that we have reassured they do not have arthritis. Time and again, worried individuals thrust x-rays into our hands and announce, "My doctor told me it was arthritis." In some cases, they are correct, but in many the label has been inappropriately applied to any number of musculoskeletal aches and pains. A sore joint or a stiff muscle does not equal arthritis. This is particularly true in younger individuals in whom arthritis is extremely uncommon. In the older person, although arthritis may exist, it is not necessarily the cause of the discomfort and may only show up through investigation as a coincidental finding. The following are some conditions that are often misconstrued as arthritis.

Neck and Back Conditions

Not all muscle or joint pain equals arthritis; similarly, not all neck and back pain is due to arthritis. Neck and back pain is an extremely common problem throughout the general population and can occur in the presence or absence of other arthritic conditions. Neck and back pain can be confusing as the pain often radiates into areas remote from the site of inflammation or injury. The complexity of the spine, the dependence of its stability on numerous muscles and ligaments, its involvement in all posture and activity, and the difficulty in resting an injured part often make neck and back pain a difficult and sometimes frustrating problem to treat.

Neck and Back Injury

The neck and the back are prone to injury. All the numerous components of the spine can be injured, ranging from a fracture of the bony portion and herniation of the disc to strains of the ligaments and muscles. The event causing the injury may be major, such as a fall from height or a motor vehicle accident, or might be so minor that the individual does not even recall a specific event and is not aware of any problem until the sudden development of pain, often 1 or 2 days later.

Pain in the neck and the back can be quite severe and incapacitating. The reasons for this are unclear. It may relate to the body's poor localization of pain in this area with subsequent radiation. It may relate to the pain caused when muscles contract to try and splint and protect the injured area. It may relate to the fact that, unlike other areas of the body, it is very difficult to rest or avoid using the spine, as it is such an integral part of posture and all movement.

Low back pain is common – 10% to 15% of individuals will experience one episode of back pain during a year and over a lifetime 80% to 90% percent of people will have at least one episode of back pain. The incidence of pain increases with age and is more common in men. The incidence of neck pain is lower and more commonly related to trauma. Low back pain is the most common cause of disability in patients under 45.

Neck and Back Strains

Strains of the neck and back generally refer to injuries to the soft tissues surrounding the spine. They are called myofascial strains; this simply refers to the tissues that are affected. It is almost impossible to localize the precise muscle or ligament that has been injured.

A myofascial strain in the neck follows a recognized or unrecognized injury. When associated with a motor vehicle accident it has been termed whiplash or whiplash associated disorder (WAD).

Definition of Whiplash Associated Disorders (WAD)

WAD I	Complaint of neck pain, stiffness or tenderness only no physical signs.
WAD II	Complaint of neck pain and musculoskeletal signs including decreased range of motion and point tenderness.
WAD III	Complaint of neck pain and neurological signs including decreased or absent deep tendon reflexes, weakness and sensory deficits.
WAD IV	Complaint of neck pain and fracture or dislocation.

Typically, in a myofascial strain there will be little if any discomfort immediately following the accident. The pain will develop anywhere from a few hours to 2 days following the injury. In cases where no specific injury is recalled, it can be quite a surprise to wake with severe neck pain and reduced mobility. The severity of the symptoms often lead an individual to fear a much more serious injury or disease than a simple sprain. The pain is not only localized to the neck: it can spread up into the head and can often be responsible for headaches. It may spread across the top of the shoulders, although it is unusual for it to progress beyond, into the arms, hands, or fingers. There may be some radiation down into the upper part of the back. There may be stiffness with reduced range of motion in the neck, making it difficult to turn the head in one direction or another. There may be quite localized tenderness to pressure, and there may be visible or palpable spasm. There may be a feeling of numbness and tingling in the hands usually affecting the little and ring finger. The reason for this is unclear, and it does not automatically mean there has been nerve damage. Medical evaluation, however, is recommended.

The lumbar or low back strain is similar to a neck strain and is generally related to trauma, although again the specific event may not be immediately apparent. Following a twisting or lifting injury or other trauma, the pain often takes many hours to develop. The reason for this is likely the time it takes to accumulate significant bruising or inflammation within the damaged tissue. As with cervical sprains, the pain is often maximal at about 48 hours following injury. The pain is generally worse in the back but can spread into the buttocks and occasionally down into the leg. There may be abnormal feeling in the lower legs and feet and possibly pins and needles, but, as with the neck, this does not always indicate nerve damage or sciatic nerve irritation (sciatica). Medical examination should rule out anything serious in these cases.

A lumbar strain can result in marked stiffness and restricted movement. The pain may be a dull ache but on certain movements there may be sudden severe sharp pain, which catches an individual unaware. Occasionally the pain is aggravated by coughing or straining, and a prolonged posture, such as standing or sitting, is uncomfortable.

Cervical or lumbar myofascial strain does not mean you have arthritis, and there is no good evidence that it leads to arthritis in the spine. It is possible that if you are an older individual and x-rays are taken of your neck or spine, these will show some degenerative arthritic changes. In the majority of cases, however, these changes have long preceded the injury and should be considered incidental findings with a principal diagnosis of a myofascial strain. In cases were the arthritis is severe, it may take a little longer than normal for the back pain to settle, and in other cases, the acute episode of back pain may be the first symptom of long-standing degeneration.

Whether or not a degree of arthritis is identified in the neck or spine, the majority of acute episodes of low back and neck pain resolve spontaneously. Among patients, 50% have settled within 1 week and over 90% are better at 2 months, although 5% to 10% unfortunately have persistent pain. In these individuals, recovery can often involve a long and frustrating course.

Mechanical or Chronic Low Back Pain

Individuals with mechanical low back pain have no identifiable systemic disease and no clearly identifiable local spinal pathology to account for their ongoing discomfort and complex of symptoms. Although these individuals constitute only a small fraction of back pain patients, they consume the largest number of resources with respect to medicine and the economy. The pain can often persist despite all treatments or interventions. In certain individuals, chronic back pain will be associated with emotional, psychological, and social problems. There is an unfortunate correlation between the development and persistence of chronic back pain and the presence of such secondary pain. A full discussion of the intricacies of chronic low back pain is beyond the scope of this book.

Within the framework of low back pain, the concept of the deconditioned spine is important to understand. The spinal structures, including ligaments and muscles, are in constant use, being involved with all posture and movement. In certain occupations, they are placed under much greater stress, such as in construction or manual labor jobs. Unfortunately, the majority of these individuals take no preventative steps in order to ensure their optimum health and fitness for the activities they endure. An Olympic athlete will undergo hours of training before attempting significant lifting maneuvers. A manual laborer is unlikely to perform even the most basic stretches before embarking on heavy physical activity. It is no surprise, therefore, that the incidence of back injury in this population is high.

The second important concept with respect to a deconditioned spine presents itself during recovery from injury. Following resolution and healing of a cervical or lumbar strain, the tissues involved in the injury lose flexibility and strength. In addition, the reduced level of activity resulting from the injury causes further deconditioning of the entire spine. Subsequently, on attempted return to activity, either through organized therapy or return to work, there is a great deal of pain and stiffness. This is interpreted by the individual as re-injury or failure of healing of the original injury and helps promote the sense of disability. Early treatment of neck or low back injuries with avoidance of prolonged rest is important in avoiding the deconditioned spine and its consequences.

Disc Herniation

The discs are the structures that sit between adjacent bones of the spine, consisting of a tough outer portion and a softer inner core. They are prone to injury, and in some cases disruption of the outer layers allows herniation of the softer inner core into the surrounding tissues. Disc herniation should not be confused with 'disc bulges'. These are often seen on special investigations, such as MRIs, and are a normal and non-significant finding. They only become significant when the bulge is substantial or indeed there has been herniation or leakage of the inner softer fluid into the region of the nervous tissue. This is what is meant by a "slipped" or herniated disc.

Herniated discs in the neck or the spine cause symptoms both locally in the form of back or neck pain, which is typically worse on bending forwards, and in the form of pain in the arms or legs. The pain radiating into the arms or legs is secondary to pressure on nerves that are emerging from the spine. This pain can be severe and burning in nature and may be associated with numbness or pins and needles. In the legs, this pain is often termed "sciatica" as it involves nerves that travel in the large nerve trunk called the sciatic nerve down the back of the leg to the foot. In severe nerve compression, there may actually be loss of power or complete loss of feeling in a certain area supplied by the nerve. The most serious of scenarios involves loss of control of bowel or bladder function when specific nerves are compressed. This is considered an emergency requiring immediate surgery.

Pain spreading into the hands or legs, even when associated with some numbness or tingling, does not necessarily signify disc herniation or nerve compression, but this should be evaluated by a physician. Even in cases were there is evidence of nerve compression, treatment is almost always non-operative in the early stages. The herniation is often associated with a great deal of inflammation, and this causes the symptoms. They often resolve if the inflammation settles. It is only in cases of progressive symptoms or persistence despite conservative measures that surgical treatment is undertaken.

Arthralgia

Literally, this means pain in a joint. While arthritis does present with arthralgia, not all arthralgia is arthritis. Arthralgia is common in such an illness as influenza, where it is transient and often moves from joint to joint. It is not associated with swelling or stiffness. Any joint in an adult that has been injured or undergone surgery may ache from time to time, often with changes in the weather. Even in cases were an adjacent bone has been broken and healed (such as the ankle joint following a shin bone or tibia fracture), this type of arthralgia can exist.

Tendonitis

This means inflammation of a tendon. Tendons are the ropes or pulleys through which muscles act. They can become inflamed for many reasons, such as acute or repetitive trauma, abnormal anatomy, or poor biomechanics. The pain can be quite severe and persistent with a quality similar to arthritis. The body has very poor localization when it comes to pain from muscles, tendons, and joints, so tendonitis is often felt as coming from the joint, which can be confused with arthritis. However, while some of the inflammatory mechanisms are the same, in general it is not arthritis and does not lead to arthritis.

Myalgia

This means pain in the muscles, which is often associated with unaccustomed exercise or, as with arthralgia, associated with influenza.

Tenosynovitis

Caused by inflammation of the sheath that surrounds a tendon, this

condition is often associated with inflammatory arthritis, such as rheumatoid arthritis, but in isolation is not a cause of arthritis. Sharp pain with
movement, crepitus, or crunching of the tendon as it glides, and local
swelling are the typical features.

Bursitis

This condition involves inflammation of a bursa, one of the many protective
sacks that occur throughout the body. The bursae are slippery sacks lined
with the same tissue that lines a joint, synovial membrane. They provide
cushioning and lubrication between structures. For example, one allows
the skin to slide easily over the bony prominences at the elbow or knee and
another cushions the rotator cuff muscles and tendons that control the
shoulder. Bursitis can result from acute or repetitive trauma. It may present
with mark swelling, often seen at the elbow or knee (for example, with
'housemaid's knee'), redness, and pain. Deeper bursae, such as those at the
shoulder or hip, present with deep pain, often intense and aggravated by
movement. In severe cases of shoulder bursitis, for example, it may be
almost impossible to move the joint due to pain. It is not uncommon for
these conditions to be confused with arthritis. Although certain joints
when affected by arthritis can show some associated bursitis, in general
bursitis is not related to arthritis.

Tennis Elbow and Similar Conditions

These conditions have many names – periostitis, apophysis, tennis and
golfer's elbow, jumper's knee (patellar tendonitis), shin splints, plantar
fasciitis (heel spurs), to name but a few. These are all conditions in which
inflammation occurs at the site of attachment of a ligament, tendon, or
muscle to bone. Partial tearing, attempted healing, and repeat injury result
in chronic inflammation with associated pain. These conditions can be
quite disabling as they often affect areas that are used frequently for daily or
work related activity. The pain is usually sharp and well localized but may
have a more diffuse, dull aching quality, with radiation down the limbs.
Many of these sites of inflammation are adjacent to joints, and the conditions are therefore often confused with arthritis. There is, however, no evidence to suggest they are related or lead to arthritis. (One exception is the
association of heel spurs and Achilles' tendonitis with psoriatic arthritis).

Chondromalacia

This refers to deterioration in the quality of the articular cartilage that overlies the end of a bone at a joint. It is most often used in reference to the degeneration that occurs on the undersurface of the kneecap (chondromalacia patellae). The condition is often associated with crunching or grinding with movement and may be associated with pain, particularly with activity. A direct look at the cartilage will reveal that instead of the smooth shiny surface there is a dull rough appearance with fissures, and on close examination, a fibrillated appearance similar to crab meat. While some of the biomechanical changes in the articular cartilage in chondromalacia are similar to those found in osteoarthritis, there is currently no clear evidence that chondromalacia leads directly to osteoarthritis. In the absence of pain, swelling or other mechanical symptoms, such as locking or giving way, simple cracking or creaking within joints does not require treatment.

Cracking Joints

Everybody's joints crack. A click or snap when moving a joint does not mean that you have osteoarthritis. It may be due to a tendon or ligament snapping across the joint or may be due to a minute vacuum creating a small bubble that bursts.

Frozen Shoulder

Also called adhesive capsulitis, this is an unusual condition in which the shoulder becomes severely painful, and then as the pain gradually settles, there is increasing stiffness with extreme immobility. The condition is more common in people with diabetes, and tends to follow trauma even to a remote part of the limb, such as a finger or wrist. There is no evidence of any inflammatory process and no evidence that it is related to or leads to osteoarthritis. The natural history for the condition is for gradual resolution over a period of 18 months to 2 years with almost complete restoration of movement and no tendency for the joints to become arthritic in later life.

DIAGNOSIS AND PROGNOSIS IN ARTHRITIS

②

Having taken a good history about your complaints, general health, family background, and many other things that may often seem quite obscure, your doctor or specialist will examine you for arthritis. This will involve a general examination with specific emphasis on the affected joint or joints. Your doctor may then decide to order some tests to evaluate your condition further. Even when arthritis is found to be the cause of the pain, you should not be frightened of the diagnosis. In most cases, the symptoms will be mild or temporary and easily treated. Progression is most often very slow and unlikely to result in significant interference in day-to-day life. The wide range of natural and traditional therapies currently available not only work preventatively but ensure that even when your arthritis does become bothersome, a solution is just around the corner.

Every arthritic joint is different. This is not only because of differences in the extent, nature, and presentation of the disease. It is also due to the fact that all patients are different. Symptoms that in one patient may not even cause them to miss a game of tennis, in others may result in substantial disability. In addition, the degree of pain and disability that a patient will tolerate before seeking attention varies greatly. To some, the inability to play a full 18 holes of golf may be a major disability, whereas others may not seek the advice of their doctor until they are practically housebound because of pain and stiffness. All these factors need to be taken into consideration and each joint treated as a separate entity.

Standard Tests

X-rays

Standard x-rays can offer a great deal of information about the bone changes around a joint. Muscles, ligaments, and cartilage are not seen unless partially crystallized, as occurs in some types of gout. Inferences can, however, often be made by examination of the anatomy and other subtle findings. The x-ray report produced by the radiologist needs to be interpreted in light of your symptoms and examination findings. Radiologists rarely have the benefit of any clinical history about the subject of the x-ray. They report all findings, and quite often comment on "arthritic" or "degenerative" changes. These may be very subtle and quite in keeping with normal findings for your age group, so do not be alarmed. Your doctor will review the films with you and let you know if there is anything serious.

There is very poor correlation between the degree of arthritis seen on x-rays and the complaints of the patient. We have seen many x-rays where the damage is so severe we wonder how the individual can get out of bed in the morning, yet the patient continues to play golf or tennis. In others, the changes are mild, yet the pain and discomfort severe. It is important to remember that orthopedic surgeons do not operate on x-rays! Regardless of what your films show, it is your symptoms that count.

Blood Tests

Blood tests are most often ordered for the evaluation of acute, severe inflammation of a joint, to rule out infection or gout. They are frequently used to evaluate the possibility of inflammatory arthritis, such as rheumatoid arthritis, psoriatic arthritis, or SLE (lupus). There are currently no blood tests for osteoarthritis.

Joint Fluid

Synovial fluid may be withdrawn from your knee with a needle to test for many different properties that may help with your diagnosis. The test is usually done in the office or clinic and should involve thorough sterilization of the skin. A small needle is used first to freeze the skin, allowing the larger needle to be introduced with minimal discomfort. The procedure is sometimes painful towards the end as the joint empties and the inflamed surfaces come into contact. A small amount of local anaesthetic may be injected into the joint at this point to reduce this sensation. The synovial fluid may have some blood in it related to the inflammation or, as often occurs following trauma, a significant amount of blood. It may be purulent as occurs in infection. Microscopic examination may reveal organisms, altered cell numbers, or crystals (as seen in gout or pseudogout). Cultures are taken if infection is suspected. The fluid is tested for sugar and proteins as well as antibodies.

Bone Scan

This test measures 'bone cell activity'. It involves injection of a (non-harmful) radioactive marker into a vein in the hand, followed, two hours later, by a scan of the whole body or a specific area. Active areas show up as 'hot spots'. Unfortunately, the test is not very specific. These hot spots can represent anything from fracture to arthritis. Care must be taken when interpreting them. We quite often get referred patients for evaluation of 'arthritis' because of a hot bone scan. Most often they have no complaints and completely normal findings at the 'hot' joint. In some cases, further investigation is required depending on the site of the hot spot, but in most cases, reassurance is all that is required. Correlation with the patient's symptoms and x-rays is essential, and in many cases, the scan is helpful in localizing pathology and directing further tests. SPECT scans work in a similar way but, like a CAT scan, can give 3-dimensional localization.

CAT Scan

A CAT scan or computer tomography uses x-rays from different angles to give a 3-dimensional image of the body. Plain x-rays are only 2-dimensional, so it is difficult to look inside structures that are superimposed. CAT scans are very helpful at looking inside joints with more detail and give excellent images of the spine. They are often better than MRI scans (see below) for looking at bony structures and arthritis.

MRI Scan

Magnetic resonance imaging uses changing magnetic fields to image the different structures in the body. Different tissues have different "resonance" properties, and these properties change if the tissue is inflamed or altered by disease. MRI provides an almost anatomy-book like picture of the body with superb detail of soft tissue, such as muscles and ligaments. It is rarely used to evaluate arthritis unless there is suspected soft tissue involvement, such as in the spine. MRI scans are extremely sensitive, and it is essential that the findings are correlated with the symptoms and clinical findings of the patient, along with other tests. Many "abnormalities" are so common as to be considered insignificant in most cases, for example, "disc bulge" in the spine and "acromio-clavicular arthritis" in the shoulder.

Specific Conditions

Arthritis in the Spine

The majority of back and neck pain is not due to arthritis, and generally resolves within a few weeks. However, in those individuals who do have persistent pain, evaluation for arthritis would involve an examination by your doctor, plain x-rays, a CAT scan, a bone scan, and possibly some blood tests to identify potential causes of the discomfort. The identification of arthritis in the spine is so common it is often hard to conclude that it is the pathology producing your pain. In certain individuals, however, a correlation can be made between symptoms and degenerative changes in the neck or back. Unfortunately, in this group, treatment options are often limited. In most people, surgical intervention is not indicated or offers less than ideal outcome with respect to pain relief. Many will wish to avoid surgery and its attendant complications. Indeed, in the absence of severe or progressive damage to the spinal cord or emerging nerves necessitating rapid intervention, surgery is considered a last resort.

Orthopedic surgeons are, in general, unable to offer much in the way of treatment unless surgery is required. Pain-killers, anti-inflammatory medicines, and perhaps physiotherapy provide a back-up, which most patients have already tried. This often leaves patients frustrated, as no one seems able to help or suggest alternatives for their care. Complementary therapies have, in our experience, been beneficial to some patients. They do not work in everyone, but, in general, have minor, if any, side effects and should therefore be considered as worthwhile treatment options.

Rheumatoid Arthritis

The diagnosis of rheumatoid arthritis can be difficult and elusive, and a referral to a rheumatologist is recommended. A careful history, examination, blood tests, and x-rays can help clarify the diagnosis. In addition, removal of fluid from a joint for testing or sampling of the joint lining and examination under the microscope can also be used to aid diagnosis if it is unclear.

In diagnosing rheumatoid arthritis, the physician will look for the following conditions:

- morning stiffness (stiffness of joints lasting at least 1 hour
     in the morning)
- 3 or more joint areas involved
- hand joints involved (wrist and knuckle joints)
- symmetrical joint involvement (same joints on both
     sides of the body)
- rheumatoid nodules (nodules under skin, generally at the elbows)
- rheumatoid factor in blood
- x-ray changes typical for rheumatoid arthritis

Much like its presentation, the course of rheumatoid arthritis is variable. Among patients, 15% to 20% run an intermittent course, showing frequent, partial, or complete remissions without the need for ongoing medical therapy. About 10% show similar long clinical remissions but require ongoing treatment. The largest group of 65% to 70% show progressive disease, which may follow a rapid or slow course. They require ongoing medical and often surgical treatment.

The outcome in rheumatoid arthritis is likely to be poor if rheumatoid factor is present in the blood tests from the outset, if rheumatoid nodules are present in the skin, or if the patient develops the disease after the age of 60. The good news is that effective and structured treatment involving a number of modalities can help slow the progress of disease, alleviate discomfort, and prolong function.

Rheumatoid arthritis is a systemic disease, and although its focus appears to be primarily in the joints, other tissues can be affected. These include the skin, where nodules can develop, usually in the forearm just below the elbow. Muscles and nerves may be affected causing weakness. The eyes can become inflamed, as can numerous other tissues, including the lung, heart, and arteries. The involvement of these other tissues is fortunately rare and associated with the more severe forms of rheumatoid arthritis.

Ankylosing Spondylitis

Diagnosis of ankylosing spondylitis relies on the characteristic symptoms, presenting in an at-risk individual, plus findings of limited spinal mobility and chest expansion, an alteration of posture, along with irritation of the sacroiliac joints. X-rays of the sacroiliac joints and the spine often reveal classic findings helping with the diagnosis of the disease. Blood tests include ESR, hemoglobin, and HLA B-27.

The outlook for ankylosing spondylitis is variable, but much better than for rheumatoid arthritis. The disease is often mild and self-limited. There is no good evidence that life expectancy is reduced. Most patients continue to function well and one-third may become pain free. For most patients the disease runs a mild course with little involvement of tissues outside the musculoskeletal system.

Psoriatic Arthropathy

The diagnosis of psoriatic arthropathy is based primarily on clinical examination and presentation. Positive blood tests are rare, as with ankylosing spondylitis, although HLA testing may be beneficial. If positive, radiographs of the spine, sacroiliac joints, or fingers may show distinctive signs of psoriatic arthritis (so-called 'pencil in cup' abnormality).

In general, psoriatic arthritis causes much less disability than rheumatoid arthritis. Only between 5% and 15% of all patients affected will progress to the severely destructive form of the arthritis with subsequent disability. Many more have a mild course with frequent remissions.

Gout and Pseudogout

The classic findings of gout in an individual with the appropriate demographics makes diagnosis relatively straightforward. It is important to differentiate the condition from acute infection, which can present in a similar manner. The other possibility is arthritis secondary to pseudogout. Confirmation is made by a combination of a blood test for uric acid and, in some cases, withdrawal of fluid from the joint and examination under the microscope for crystals.

The diagnosis for pseudogout is based on the patient's demographics, the clinical findings, the presence of calcium deposits on x-ray, and the presence of crystals in fluid taken from the joint. As opposed to gout (negatively birefringent), the crystals seen in pseudogout are positively birefringent.

In general, the prognosis for most individuals following an attack of gout is excellent. Once the acute attack has resolved, treatment, including changes to diet and medications, is very effective at preventing recurrence.

Acute Bacterial or Septic Arthritis

The diagnosis of acute bacterial arthritis is based on careful evaluation of risk factors, including recent systemic infection, history of diabetes, history of inflammatory arthritis, recent trauma or surgical intervention, locally or elsewhere in the body, and the presence of a joint replacement. Monitoring of temperature is important, and blood tests may be taken to reveal raised white cell count and ESR and occasionally culture of organisms from the blood.

Fluid can be drained from the joint; it is often thick and yellow with small clots within it. This is in contrast to normal joint fluid, which is straw colored and clear and may be present in increased amounts in normal arthritis or following trauma. The fluid is tested for the presence of organisms and the culture of organisms. It is also checked for crystals, as other diagnoses with this presentation can be gout or pseudogout or acute inflammatory arthritis. The number of white cells in the fluid is important.

The diagnosis of bacterial or septic arthritis may be difficult as cultures are often negative. In these cases, a high index of suspicion must be maintained and the most aggressive form of treatment embarked upon. The inflammatory process in the joint caused by the bacteria produces enzymes and chemicals that are destructive to bone and cartilage, and damage has been noted as early as 48 hours after the onset of infection.

X-rays of the joint are generally not helpful apart from revealing the fluid within the joint. If the infection is not treated and becomes destructive, erosions around the joint and loss of bone substance can be noted as early as 7 to 14 days.

Early identification of septic arthritis along with aggressive treatment, including surgical drainage and antibiotics, ensures, in most cases, a successful outcome with an essentially normal joint once the inflammation and stiffness have resolved.

Infection of the small skin incisions following arthroscopy does not constitute a joint infection. Generally, only oral antibiotics are required, but the patient should be monitored carefully.

Treatment Plans

Early treatment of all forms of arthritis is important with regard to slowing progression of the disease. Your family doctor will have the expertise to evaluate you and plan treatment. This may involve referral to a specialist, usually a rheumatologist or an orthopedic surgeon. Rheumatologists treat all forms of arthritis and specialize in the evaluation and diagnosis of the many diffuse inflammatory conditions, such as rheumatoid arthritis, SLE, and psoriatic arthritis. They plan medical treatment, including physiotherapy, occupational therapy, medication, and injection therapy. Apart from a small number performing simple office diagnostic arthroscopy, they do not perform surgery.

Your naturopathic doctor can play an important complementary role in the treatment of all forms of arthritis. A naturopath will evaluate your overall medical condition as it relates to your arthritis and institute a course of therapy aimed at reducing symptoms and progression of the disease, promoting the body's own healing potential, and reducing the side effects of other medications.

Orthopedic surgeons assess and treat arthritis with emphasis on joint damage. Referral to an orthopedic surgeon does not mean you are going to have surgery. Apart from certain emergencies, such as an infected joint, surgery is a last resort. Your orthopedist will ensure that all other appropriate non-surgical therapies have been tried before recommending an operation. Even then, the decision to go ahead is yours. The orthopedic surgeon will explain the available options, benefits and risks, and will allow you to come to an informed decision.

Naturopathic medicine can be useful even if it is decided that surgery is required. Naturopathic supplementation and therapies can be employed to prepare the body for surgery and maximize healing. The same supplements that are used to repair cartilage can be used pre- and post-operatively to prevent further destruction of the joint. Dietary changes, such as increased ingestion of protein and zinc, are also useful to promote more rapid and effective wound healing. In addition, homeopathics, such as arnica, can be used pre- and post-operatively to help reduce pain and inflammation. A few of these therapies may interfere with medications or surgery, so discussion with your naturopathic doctor is advised if surgery is being planned.

Although treatment of rheumatoid arthritis has some similarities with osteoarthritis, in general the regimes are very different. The reason for this relates not only to the wide range syndromes associated with rheumatoid arthritis, but also to its nature as a systemic disease involving the immune system and extensive inflammation. Although treatment should always be individualized, this is most important in rheumatoid arthritis where variations in presentation, progression, and severity need to be matched with the individual's personal characteristics.

Education

A well-informed patient can understand and thereby cooperate in the healing process, but it is estimated that on average, patients remember only 10% of what is told to them at a meeting with their doctor. For the doctor, this 10% needs to be key 'healing' information that does not cause undue fear or anxiety. Important points need to be emphasized repeatedly, and if possible, included in a simple handout that can be taken away by patients for later perusal. The patient can participate in this education process by writing down information and posing questions to be asked at the next appointment so that these issues may be addressed.

One set of explanations is not going to work for everyone. Patients have vastly different expectations with regards to the knowledge that they require and vastly different abilities with regard to the knowledge they can understand and assimilate. Again, every patient needs to be considered individually.

PHYSICAL TREATMENTS FOR ARTHRITIS

③

P hysical treatments for arthritis are applied to the affected area to reduce pain and improve function. They include ice, heat, massage, and acupuncture, among others. Many of these treatments can be administered on your own and used effectively in your management of arthritis. Others are used by therapists as part of their therapeutic regimen.

Rest

Resting of a joint, often with use of a splint provided by an occupational therapist, can be very useful in allowing an acutely inflamed joint to settle. There seems to be a direct correlation between joint movement and involvement in rheumatoid arthritis. This modality needs to be carefully monitored so as not to induce stiffness or deconditioning (reduced muscle tone and strength).

Ice Treatments

Ice treatment, cooling, or cryotherapy is a widely used modality for the treatment of pain and inflammation, particularly following injury. Ice can also be used to treat acute inflammation of a joint, particularly in an acute flare of osteoarthritis and crystal arthritis, rheumatoid or other inflammatory arthritis.

The benefits of ice application are numerous. Ice application to the skin has been shown to decrease skin, intra-muscular, and joint temperature. Cooling of nerves reduces muscle spasm and pain. There is a direct affect on the local inflammatory response. The local metabolic rate is reduced and the permeability of blood vessels decreased. The effects last after removal of the ice, and there is no evidence that it causes a reactive increase in blood flow later on.

The most effective form of ice therapy is wet ice. Crushed ice in a plastic bag wrapped in a wet towel applied to the skin for approximately 20 minutes is the most efficient way of reducing tissue temperature. The most convenient form is probably a re-useable 'gel' cold pack. These last about 15 to 20 minutes. Caution is recommended when applying these packs directly to skin. Normally, they should be wrapped within a light towel.

Cold packs can usually be applied for 10 to 20 minutes – it is unusual for applications under 30 minutes to cause injury. The risk increases if ice or gel packs are applied directly to skin. In general, it is safest to have them wrapped in a thin towel. This minimizes the possibility of frostbite. Any numbness or tingling should be an indicator to remove the pack immediately. Upon removal of the pack, an interval of 40 minutes to one hour should be allowed before reapplication.

Superficial Heat Treatments

Besides the psychological effect of comfort, heat has a number of beneficial effects on joints and tissues. It induces muscle relaxation and reduces spasm. It increases the flexibility of tissues with a direct effect on the properties of collagen. Heat increases the metabolism of tissues, improves blood supply, and relieves pain. Superficial heat allows penetration through the skin, superficial tissues, and upper layers of muscle. Deeper tissues and joints are reached by heat from ultrasound and diathermy.

Superficial heat is generally applied through heat packs, heating blankets, and, particularly in the case of hand therapy, paraffin wax baths. Superficial heat should not be used during the acute stages of inflammation.

For example, a joint that has been recently injured or had an acute flare of arthritis should initially be treated with ice.

Superficial heat, although often feeling more comfortable, has potential to increase inflammation and swelling. It should not be used during an acute flare-up of gout or any of the other inflammatory arthritides. Superficial heat is ideal, however, at all other times for the treatment of pain and stiffness associated with arthritis. There is no evidence that superficial heat increases the severity or progression of rheumatoid arthritis.

Ultrasound

Deep heat is probably the most important effect of ultrasound. Ultrasound is mechanical energy in the form of high frequency vibrations, which are transmitted to the tissues. Ultrasound is applied to the skin through a hand-held device and conductive gel. It has mechanical properties that may alter nerve receptor sensitivity, reducing spasm in muscle and decreasing pain. It may also promote a healing response in cells by improving protein synthesis. Ultrasound is particularly useful in the treatment of muscle and tendon injuries.

Although benefits such as increased extensibility, blood flow, decreased joint stiffness, muscle spasm, and pain are reported from ultrasound treatment, it may be contraindicated in some arthritic conditions where deep tissue heating can accelerate joint destruction. However, ultrasound in the lower, non-thermal energy levels (30mW/cm2) has been shown to promote fracture healing and promote cartilage repair.

Non-Thermal Effects
– tissue regeneration
– soft tissue repair
– increased protein synthesis
– reduced swelling
– decreased pain and spasm

Thermal Effects
– increased metabolic rate and enzyme activity
– increased blood flow

– increased flexibility of collagen and muscle
– decreased sensitivity of neuro-receptors

Contrast Treatment

This treatment involves the combination of heat and cold. Besides the effects of heat and cold noted above, contrast baths are particularly effective at reducing tissue swelling. Generally, a combination of 3 to 4 minutes warm followed by 1 minute cold over 3 cycles is recommended.

Short-Wave Diathermy

Diathermy involves passage of a high frequency current with no nerve stimulation. A rapid vibration induces deep heat in the tissues. The effect is similar to that of ultrasound. It should not be used near metal implants or in the presence of heart pacemakers. It is generally contraindicated, as with other deep heating modalities, for the treatment of arthritis.

Interferential Bio Electrical Stimulation

This treatment involves the application of two "interfering" medium frequency alternating currents. The interference results in the production of variable intensity current within the tissues. This is applied through pads or suction cups and results in bioelectric stimulation without significant heating. Beneficial effects include pain relief, control of swelling, reduced muscle wasting, improved flexibility, and muscle strength.

Hydrotherapy

Hydrotherapy is the external use of water-based modalities for treatment. One of the most obvious and frequently used benefits of water for the patient with arthritis is the ability to exercise without significant strain on the joint. Water-based activity does not involve any impact loading and subsequently allows exercise of joints, such as the hips and knees, without causing pain or further injury. Water provides variable resistance to movement depending on speed and is therefore ideal for allowing individuals to pace themselves.

Whirlpool baths can be used, depending on their temperature, to provide heat, cyrotherapy, or contrast bath treatments. Whirlpools should be avoided for the first 2 weeks following surgery due to the slight increase in risk of infection.

Physiotherapy

Physiotherapists play an extremely valuable role in the care of the arthritic patient, whether for prevention, treatment of active disease, or recovery from surgery. Physiotherapy incorporates the education of the patient about an injury or disease process, discussion of their expectations, and guidance and precautions with regards to activity. Physical therapy incorporates passive and active stretching, strengthening, mobilization, posture, and balance, as well as instruction on how to exercise and use joints without causing damage.

Exercise is important in maintaining joint mobility and muscle strength. Weight-bearing exercise is also beneficial in maintaining bone density, which often deteriorates in rheumatoid arthritis.

Occupational Therapy

Occupational therapy, like physiotherapy, plays a pivotal role in the treatment and management of arthritis. A physiotherapist may work closely with an occupational therapist with respect to posture and ergonomics (teaching correct and safe techniques for tasks at home and in the workplace). Occupational therapy is also involved with splinting and the provision or adaptation of devices that enable easy functioning.

Occupational therapists are involved in patient education, particularly with reference to daily activity. Activity modification involves pacing and postural retraining to minimize discomfort and maximize function. Recommending and providing mechanical aids is an aspect of the OT's work that is extremely varied. It extends from provision of a simple cane through devices such as large grip cutlery, extended devices for allowing socks and stockings to be applied, tools for reaching, twisting, and turning, and devices in the home as varied as a hand grip in the bathroom to motorized chairs. Splinting is another important role. The design and manufacture of splints for joints to provide rest or support is extremely valuable in arthritis.

Cane

This simple walking aid is an extremely valuable and under-utilized tool in the treatment of arthritis in the lower extremities. This should be used in the hand opposite to the leg that is most affected. In the hip, it can reduce forces across the hip by almost 50% and thus can relieve significant pain.

Bracing

Braces are devices applied to a joint or body part to provide support by improving stability and function. A brace may be as simple as an elastic bandage or slip-on elastic sleeve. While these devices do not provide sub-stantial physical support or help with instability, they do help control swelling, provide heat, and increase sensory feedback from the joint.

Technology has advanced considerably with respect knee braces. In recent years, numerous arthritis braces have been developed. These custom-made braces apply pressure across the knee in order to unload the area of the joint that is painful from the arthritis. In some cases, a trial with an off-the-shelf brace of a similar type is allowed in order to assess whether the individual is likely to gain any benefit from this type of brace.

Orthotics

Orthotics, in their simplest form, are inserts within footwear designed to aid the foot during walking. Behind this simple statement lies a great deal of conflicting opinion within the medical community, and podiatry in partic-ular, as to their role in the treatment of arthritic conditions. Orthotics acts on the foot directly, but can have influence on the biomechanics of the entire leg, with potentially beneficial effect on the ankle, knee, hip, and spine.

The orthotic represents only part of an overall treatment plan. It does not in itself represent a sole form of treatment and should be undertaken in conjunction with other treatment modalities, including those from other medical specialists, in order to achieve optimal effect.

Due to the very nature of the disease process, the orthotic should be adjustable to allow for changes as they occur and to ensure that a 'flexible prescription' is achieved. By this it is meant that the orthotic is not acting on the foot too aggressively, leading to trauma (both to soft tissue and joint) that aggravates inflammation and thereby increases discomfort. Effective, ongoing, and timely communication with the prescribing foot specialist is important. The need for adjustments to the orthotic is common in arthritic cases.

Yoga

Yoga is a type of exercise that employs both the body and the mind. Its purpose is to bring a sense of balance to the body, mentally and physically, so that the body may be in the best possible position to heal. Yoga itself does not create health, but instead helps to provide an environment that allows the body to function optimally.

Yoga is best known as a physical practice. It utilizes gentle stretching, breathing, and relaxation techniques. Each of these techniques follows a specific pattern or sequence that helps to relax the mind and energize the body. It begins with concentration on breathing. Focusing on the breath helps to quiet the mind. When the mind is quiet, the release of cortisol, our stress hormone, decreases. There next follows a series of gentle movements and poses that help to strengthen and lengthen the muscles. This also helps to increase the circulation through the body, which in turn provides new nutrients to damaged or inflamed areas of the body, and helps sweep away metabolic by-products.

The benefit of yoga exercises to musculo-skeletal disorders has been clinically put to the test. In a study involving patients with osteoarthritis of the hands, the application of yoga was observed. Such symptoms as pain, strength, motion, joint circumference, and hand function were followed. Over an 8-week period, patients either received a yoga program once a week or no therapy at all. The group treated with yoga showed significant improvement over the control group during the 8 weeks, particularly for pain during activity and finger range of motion.

It appears that through the use of gentle stretching, deep breathing, and relaxation, a positive effect can be achieved with respect to osteoarthritis and other musculoskeletal disorders. Whether due to a decrease in the stress hormone cortisol, itself an inflammatory agent, or to an improved harmony between the body and mind, yoga is a useful treatment modality. Some caution is advised in the presence of a total hip replacement, and this should be discussed with your surgeon.

Massage

Massage has long been used as a technique for controlling pain. Defined as the treatment of disease or injury through the manual manipulation of body tissues, massage is employed for the relief of pain and spasm, to induce relaxation, to stretch and break down scarring and adhesions, and to increase circulation and metabolism. Massage promotes the resorption and metabolism of toxins and the residua of inflammation. The basic movements include efflcurage, petrissage, friction, tapotement, and vibration.

There are several ways in which massage is thought to relieve pain. One involves the blocking of painful stimuli. Pain is felt when sensors in the skin, muscles, joints, and other tissues are stimulated. These sensors send messages through nerve fibers to the brain where the sensation is interpreted. The theory is that massage gently stimulates adjacent fibers, sending another set of messages to the brain. This acts almost like an overload on the system and not all of the messages get to the brain. As the massage is 'new' or 'different' to the more constant pain of arthritis, the arthritis pain is felt less, even though the massage is not actually painful.

Massage has also been shown to stimulate the release of enkephalins and endorphins, the body's natural painkillers. These hormones act on the same receptors as powerful drugs, such as morphine, reducing the awareness and intensity of pain.

Massage helps to increase local circulation, improving the flow of nutrients to an area, thereby increasing the amount of available material for healing. An increase in circulation will also help to remove the inflammatory chemicals, which not only contribute to further inflammation, but can act as free radical stimulators that hinder healing.

As most people have experienced, when a joint is injured in any way, the surrounding muscles and tissue usually become quite stiff and sore. The same is true with arthritis. Massage can be very useful in helping to loosen those tissues and increase the mobility and range of motion of each joint.

The benefits of massage have been tested clinically. One such study looked at 2 groups of elderly nursing home residents suffering from chronic arthritis pain. Over a 36-week period, trained staff massaged patients regularly. Pain scores were evaluated at the end of the trial. The results showed that pain had dissipated in each of the involved patients. A decrease in anxiety was also seen, most likely brought about by the combination of a decrease in pain and the feeling of relaxation that massage induces. When levels of stress and anxiety are diminished, there is a drop in inflammatory hormones produced. This in itself helps to decrease pain and increase healing.

Contraindications are few. Following acute injury or a severe flare up of arthritis, or in the presence of an open wound, local massage would not be advisable in that area.

Magnets

The use of magnets or magnetotherapy stems back to Cleopatra's time. It is said that she used to sleep with a magnet under her to prevent or slow the aging process. Since then magnets have been used in various ways. The first recorded therapeutic magnet came from material called magnetite. This is a substance found in the earth with a weak magnetic charge. The substance was then crushed and made into a paste and applied as a poultice to an injured area.

There are several theories as to how magnets may work to alleviate pain and inflammation. One theory employs the nature of the pain signal itself. It is believed that a pain signal when transmitted across a cell depolarizes that cell. Magnets are thought to raise the threshold for depolarization on a cellular level. This would then prevent the cell from depolarizing easily, and therefore prevent the transmission of pain across it.

It is also believed that injured tissue produces a positive charge. Thus if the negative end of a magnet is placed over the tissue, a natural balance of charge is re-established. This is thought to improve circulation, allowing blood vessels to dilate and provide more nutrients to the area.

Several studies have been conducted to determine the efficacy of magnets as a form of treatment for musculoskeletal injuries or diseases. One double-blind placebo-controlled study took a look at the effect of magnets on arthritis. This study confirmed the relief of arthritic pain through the use of magnets without any adverse side effects. Another double-blind placebo-controlled study evaluated pulsed magnet fields on 37 patients with osteoarthritis in either the knee or the hip. The treatments lasted 30 minutes each and were performed on average 4 times a week. At the end of the study, 39% of the patients receiving the real magnet therapy reported reduction in pain. Only 8% of the placebo group reported a drop in pain. Although more extensive studies need to be performed into the exact mechanism and efficacy of magnets as a therapy for arthritis or other musculoskeletal problems, there appears to be some value to the this treatment modality.

There have been no adverse reactions reported, but there are some situations where magnets should not be used. Magnetotherapy or magnets themselves should not be use in pregnant women. Although it is unclear if there is any effect on the fetus, and until it is known for certain that it is safe during pregnancy, it is best to avoid it all together. In addition, those individuals with pace-makers or any other electrical device inside the body should avoid all types of magnet therapy. The change in polarization from the magnet may alter the function of the device.

Acupuncture

Acupuncture is a therapeutic method for promoting natural healing of the body through the insertion of needles. Traditional Chinese Medicine teaches that there are a series of 12 energy channels that run through the body, known as meridians. These meridians are somewhat like blood vessels and nerves in that they are the route through which energy is dispersed and nutrients are delivered throughout the body. Much as a defect in an artery or nerve causes pain, inflammation, swelling and other pathology, so does an obstruction in a meridian. Energy in Traditional Chinese Medicine is called Qi. It is this Qi that circulates through the meridians and heals the body.

There are hundreds of specific points along these meridians. Each point acts like a reservoir of potential energy for that meridian. If there is a block or problem in the meridian, by stimulating a certain point or points, the energy can be released and flow restored. This helps to heal the meridian and to re-establish a beneficial flow of energy though the body.

Although acupuncture is relatively new to the Western world, it has been used therapeutically in Asia for over 2000 years. It was not until the 1970s that physicians from the United States traveled to China to observe and learn acupuncture first hand. Subsequently, several studies were performed in an attempt to discover the mechanism behind pain relief through needle insertion. It was then shown that endogenous opioids or endorphins were released upon needle insertion. Since these studies, the acceptance and use of acupuncture in Western society has grown immensely. The Westernized scientific description of acupuncture is a stimulation of the nervous system by inserting a needle into the body. This stimulation causes a release in specific chemical substances that influence the muscles, spine, and brain. These various chemicals then bring about a relief in pain, a decrease in inflammation, or a balance back to the body.

Musculoskeletal pain is probably the area where acupuncture is used most widely in our society. One study looked at the difference between acupuncture versus exercise as a treatment for osteoarthritis. Thirty-two patients waiting for total hip replacements were randomly divided into 2 groups. Group A had 6 acupuncture sessions lasting 25 minutes each, while group B, the control group, was given advice and exercises for the hip to be performed over the 6 weeks. The symptoms assessed were pain and function. At the end of the 6 weeks, improvement was found in group A, while no significant improvement was seen in group B. This study confirmed the hypothesis that acupuncture is more effective than exercise in the relief of arthritic symptoms. Other studies have shown similar results. Upon amalgamation of 7 trials, 393 patients with arthritis in the knee were examined for pain and function. According to the trials performed, there was strong evidence that acupuncture was effective in pain relief for osteoarthritis. A National Institutes of Health panel in the United States concluded in 1997 that there was sufficient evidence to support the use of acupuncture in osteoarthritis and low back pain. Acupuncture may be used to relieve pain, reduce muscle spasm, and improve mobility in back pain due to arthritis. We have found it to be particularly useful in the relief of radiating 'nerve pain' which spreads into the arms or legs.

There are usually no side effects with acupuncture. Because acupuncture involves the movement of hormones, steroids, and natural chemicals in the body to promote healing, very few adverse reactions have taken place. However, there can be an initial flare of symptoms before the relief. You should not be alarmed by this reaction because it is considered a sign that things are changing in the body for the better. This reaction should not last past the first few treatments. If pain persists, stop the treatments and consult your therapist.

There is very little pain on the insertion of the needle. A small pinprick sensation may be felt as the needle passes through the top layers of the skin, which are laden with nerve endings. Once past these layers, there are usually no sharp sensations. Some people feel a pressure or a heavy feeling around the needle. This, too, is considered a positive effect, an indicator that the treatment will be effective.

Acupuncture needles are very thin and are solid, unlike hypodermic needles that are hollow in order to take blood or deliver a drug to the body. As they are so small, they rarely leave any trace of their presence. There is usually no blood or other markings after the needle is withdrawn.

There is no problem with receiving acupuncture while on any pharmaceutical or natural medications. The acupuncture treatment will not alter the efficacy of the drug or supplement. The only place to be careful with acupuncture is during pregnancy. Many of the points have been shown to stimulate uterine contractions, so it is best to refrain from acupuncture during pregnancy.

Chiropractic

Chiropractic care may be helpful in the relief of pain in arthritis. However, like most other forms of arthritic therapies, chiropractic treatment is dependant on the type and stage of arthritis.

Chiropractic manipulation is the gentle movement of joints and the surrounding musculature. The movement is often small and may be associated with a 'pop', thought to be a release of carbon dioxide in the joint. The theory behind chiropractic manipulation is that when a joint becomes 'fixated', it can impart neurologic and biomechanical impairment, increasing irritation and inflammation. Chiropractic manipulation of fixated joints or spinal segments aims to improve biomechanical and neurological function by restoring normal motion, relaxing tight muscles, and improving joint coordination. An arthritic joint results in decreased motion and increased fixation. Chiropractic care can increase the mobility of a joint, helping to relieve the associated stiffness of arthritis.

Chiropractic manipulation can be useful in the earlier stages of arthritis. However, it is generally not appropriate in late-stage arthritis where the joint is weakened, deformed, and demonstrates considerable loss of motion. Manipulation in this instance may increase pain or inflammation. Similarly, chiropractic manipulation is contraindicated in the presence of acute inflammation and is therefore rarely indicated in rheumatoid or other inflammatory forms of arthritis. Caution is to be exercised in manipulation of the neck in arthritis due to the possibility of segment instability.

Despite its widespread acceptance and use by the public, there remains little in the way of clinical studies to support the role of chiropractic care in the treatment of back pain due to arthritis. We have both encountered patients who have found relief through chiropractic modalities, and in the absence of contraindications to its use, such as neurologic deficit or compromise, it remains a relatively safe form of therapy. Knowledgeable registered chiropractors will let you know if they feel treatment is advisable or likely to be beneficial. In general, some effect should be noted within 3 to 4 visits.

Chiropractic philosophy suggests that spinal manipulation may be beneficial in the prevention of arthritis. However, no clinical evidence is available to support this theory. While there are some studies confirming a role for chiropractic treatment in back pain, there is no clinical data supporting a specific role in arthritis.

DIETARY TREATMENTS FOR ARTHRITIS

(4)

The primary factor when considering diet and arthritis is weight. Excess weight increases stress on the weight-bearing joints and has been correlated with the development and progression of arthritis. Thus, most diets that reduce body weight have been shown to be beneficial in the treatment of arthritis of the weight-bearing joints (hips, knees, and ankles). Weight loss can also be considered a preventative measure to avoid development of the condition. There is a definite link between obesity and the development of osteoarthritis. A good example is the fact that the kneecap transmits about 5 times your body weight when climbing stairs. Every pound you lose is therefore 5 pounds off your kneecap!

In addition to weight loss, there are specific foods that will directly increase or decrease both inflammation and pain within an arthritic joint. Certain foods can cause allergic inflammatory symptoms in some people. There are specific foods that have this effect more so than others. Some foods, such as animal products, including milk and meat, directly increase the production of inflammatory products, such as prostaglandins. By increasing the consumption of these foods, one may experience an increase in pain and inflammation in the joint. We have seen this many times with our patients. However, it is important to note that all people react differently. Some arthritic individuals are very sensitive and will notice a great change by either increasing or decreasing certain foods. Others are less sensitive and will barely notice a difference with a change in diet. Like all forms of treatment, in any disease, not all therapies have the same effect on each person.

Weight Loss and Maintenance Diets

Weight loss is the most powerful dietary therapy for arthritis available. Not only will it decrease the stress on each joint during activity, it will also help many other areas in the body. It will help to reduce cholesterol, improve the strength of the heart and circulatory system, prevent diabetes, and increase energy. Weight loss is the simplest therapy to introduce and the most cost effective.

Many different 'diets' have been developed over time to try to slow down or stop our ever-growing weight problem. Diet trends come and go, but, despite varying degrees of initial success, the calorie-deprivation, low-fat, and high-carbohydrate programs have *not* been shown to be consistently effective over time. Even the latest high-protein diets have some serious shortcomings.

Diet Trends

Calorie-reduced diets flaunt their rapid weight loss, in some cases up to 5 pounds each week. This type of weight loss, however, causes other problems, which make maintenance of the reduced weight very difficult. Excessively rapid weight loss stimulates production of an enzyme known as lipoprotein lipase, which forces our bodies to store more fat. Ultimately, this slows down our metabolic rate and therefore slows down weight loss. These diets at this stage mimic starvation and force the body to hold onto whatever food it is given. As well, the food groups chosen in these diets are imbalanced and disproportionately high in carbohydrates.

With the advent of the low-fat diet came the theory that if you want to lose fat, don't eat it! Dean Ornish's diet is one such low fat diet. Not only is this diet difficult to follow due to its nutritional restrictions, but the extreme reduction in fat leaves individuals permanently hungry. It may

also have a detrimental effect on the body. While low fat diets are very successful in lowering LDL ('bad cholesterol') levels, they also reduce HDL
('good cholesterol') levels quite dramatically. Certain studies show that
these low fat diets may even *increase* the risk of heart disease by lowering
HDL levels too far. If you eliminate all the foods with fat in them, all that
is left are grains, fruits, and vegetables, essentially another version of a
high-carbohydrate diet that, as we shall see, will eventually fail. Removing
'good' unsaturated fats from our diet is also dangerous for our health, for
these fats are integral to the construction of cell membranes and the regulation of hormones, among other essential bodily functions.

Eating just a diet high in carbohydrates seems to be a logical solution
to our weight-loss problem. These ingested carbohydrates are low in fat,
low in cholesterol, and therefore lower in calories. So it seems to make
sense to eat carbohydrates primarily, such as pasta, rice, or potatoes, a
regime promoted by *Fit for Life* and the Canada Food Guide, for example.
Unfortunately, once the carbohydrates are ingested, this picture almost
reverses due to the different hormonal secretion that occurs in response to
a high carbohydrate meal. There is, in fact, an increase in fat production
and storage as well as a rise in blood triglyceride and cholesterol levels.
These plain and simple carbohydrates become havoc-reeking substrates
that damage the body. Sadly, this diet was advocated before any sound clin
ical data was collected. On paper, these foods looked good, but in reality
they have only increased our weight problem, accentuating the process of
fat storage that we are now trying to reverse. A high carbohydrate diet has
also increased our risk of diet-related diseases.

In a study of the French population, who have far less obesity and cardiovascular disease than North Americans, Dr Michel Montignac was one
of the first to postulate that carbohydrate, rather than fat, is the crucial
component in weight gain. He also questioned the effect of low calorie
diets. Montignac's suggestion that the secretion of insulin could be tightly
controlled simply by consuming only those carbohydrates with a low
glycemic (sugar) index inspired Dr Morrison Bethea, Head of Cardiac
Surgery at Mercy-Baptist Hospital in New-Orleans, to conduct studies on
the insulin-cholesterol connection. By following a diet consisting of low
glycemic carbohydrates, total cholesterol levels were reduced by 20% to
30% in most individuals. Dr Jennifer Marks at the University of Miami

performed another series of studies on insulin resistance. She recognized that insulin resistance was characterized by glucose intolerance, an increase in cholesterol and triglycerides, high blood pressure, and obesity. It is well known that any one of these conditions alone greatly increases the risk of heart disease. However, further studies showed that the risk increased dramatically in the presence of more than one condition. This was demonstrated by a PROCAM (Prospective Cardiovascular Munster) study of 2,754 men between the ages of 40 and 60: if a person had diabetes *or* high blood pressure alone, then the risk of a heart attack was 2.5 times greater than that of a normal individual, but when an individual had both diabetes and high blood pressure, the risk increased 8 times. Dr David Brown has shown that excessive insulin levels stimulate growth of the cells lining arteries, which, in turn, decreases the available space for the blood to flow. This ultimately increases blood pressure. High insulin levels also instruct the kidneys to hold onto salt, again increasing blood pressure.

If high-carbohydrate diets are so ineffective and potentially dangerous, what about the new protein diets? The focus of many of the high-protein diets is simply to lose weight, quickly. They are not concerned with what type of weight is lost as long as a reduction is seen on the scales. Unfortunately, much of the loss is from muscle rather than fat, but maintaining muscle in the body is essential for permanent weight loss. Muscle cells contain components called mitochondria, which can be considered the 'calorie furnaces' or 'power houses' for the body. These cells burn up fat and create more energy. The more muscle you have, the more fat burning potential exists. Despite the potential for being effective in reducing weight in the short term, these protein diets are often so complex that the average person finds them too difficult to follow for any length of time. In addition, some are so restrictive of other food groups or imbalanced that they impose a separate set of problems, such as ketosis, which can damage the kidneys.

Several high protein diets have become popular. Programs such as the Carbohydrate Addict's Diet advocated by Rachael and Richard Heller, Dr Atkins' New Diet, and the Protein Power Plan diet developed by Michael and Mary Eades are biochemically well-grounded. Their premise of reducing insulin secretion so that we do not store our food as fat is sound. While they provide a foundation on which to build an effective protein-based diet, they lack many nutrients and are quite deficient in valuable carbohydrates, such as fruits and vegetables. These nutrients are vital to the growth and well-being of the body. In addition, if the carbohydrate content of the diet is too low in relation to protein, the body will assume a starvation state called ketosis. This process is essentially the body's emergency response to lack of food. Its purpose is survival at the expense of health. Ketosis results in symptoms such as nausea, dehydration, light-headedness, and bad breath. Toxic effects to the body include kidney damage. Ketosis may be fatal to diabetics and to the fetus in pregnancy.

With respect to weight reduction, ketosis results in weight loss due to dehydration and loss of muscle tissue. Not only is this harmful to the body but ultimately causes increased weight gain. Protein ingestion in ketosis can stimulate insulin release to convert the amino acids into fat. Also studies have shown that ketogenic diets alter fat cells to make them more hungry for fat storage.

Compliance with many of the protein diets is low due to their dietary restrictions. The Atkins' Diet outlaws condiments and dressings, leaving the allowable food quite bland. Both the Atkins' Diet and the Protein Power Plan involve complex measurements and calculations that are difficult to follow. The average busy individual has only 30 minutes to prepare and eat a meal. The Carbohydrate Addict's Diet offers a reward meal every day, which not only slows the weight loss process but makes dieters feel as if they are being deprived all day long so that a "reward" is then needed. A program of deprivation followed by reward is not a healthy approach to weight loss maintenance, nor likely to result in a lifelong dietary change. Barry Sear's The Zone is a good *maintenance* diet, but it can take many months to see any significant weight loss.

The Naturopathic Diet

In order to achieve healthy and permanent weight loss, it is important not simply to deprive ourselves of fat or calories. What we need is a relatively simple and convenient diet that enables immediate weight loss and long-term weight management without potential damage to our health. The "naturopathic" diet we have developed in our medical practice achieves these goals by training our body to use food as fuel rather than storing it as fat, leading to permanent weight loss and increasing our energy level. This is achieved with simple changes rather than with rigid dietary restrictions, in two stages, the weight loss stage, which adopts many of the clinically proven elements of popular protein diets, and the weight maintenance stage, which restores a truly natural balance to the diet.

The Hypoglycemia-Hyperglycemia Connection

The key factor in a clinically sound and effective weight loss program is the control of a substance called insulin. Insulin is a hormone secreted by the pancreas. Its chief role is to keep blood sugar within a certain range. If the blood sugars get too high, insulin is produced to bring them back down. It does this by promoting removal of sugar from the blood and its storage as glycogen or fat. The other main hormone involved in blood sugar control is glucagon. This hormone is responsible for increasing blood sugars when they get too low. Together, insulin and glucagon maintain optimum blood sugar levels and stores for various metabolic demands.

*Hypo*glycemia is a condition in which blood glucose levels are abnormally low. This often occurs in reaction to *hyper*glycemia or high sugar levels following a high carbohydrate meal. After the ingestion of carbohydrates the breakdown of food into sugar is quite rapid. This sugar is then delivered to the blood and glucose levels rise. The faster the breakdown of food into sugar, the faster the delivery of sugar and the higher the blood sugar levels rise. Due to the fact that the simple building blocks of carbohydrates are sugars and the bonds between them are weak relative to that of protein, a large amount of glucose is formed and delivered quickly to the blood after a meal rich in carbohydrates. It is here that insulin is called upon to scoop up all this sugar and carry it out of the blood. Glycogen stores are full and it is therefore deposited as fat.

A few hours later, most of this meal has been stored as fat and our blood sugar levels are now too low, causing hypoglycemia. Our body senses this and we feel very tired, dizzy, and possibly nauseated. Then your body begins to crave foods that will release sugar into the blood quickly, such as a sweet treat or a starch. It is a rare individual who craves a piece of chicken when they are hypoglycemic! Most of us indulge in carbohydrates, once again raising our blood-sugar levels and starting the whole process anew. If you find that by 10:00 a.m. or 3:00 p.m. you are tired and hungry, take a look at your diet. Your breakfast or lunch was probably high in carbohydrates, creating this problem.

Insulin Resistance

Most North Americans have grown up on a diet that is high in carbo-hydrates. Cereal or toast for breakfast, a sandwich for lunch, and pasta for dinner. Over the years our insulin-glucagon system has been over-worked to the point of insensitivity. Our hormone responses have become exaggerated in order to achieve the same effect. Approximately 3 out of 4 Americans have a slight to serious problem with their blood-sugar level control mechanisms. This is known as insulin resistance, where there is a decreased reaction to insulin output, thereby stimulating extra insulin release. This extra insulin in our blood (hyperinsulinemia) acts as a barrier to using the existing fat in our bodies by blocking access to it.

If we need glucose or energy and cannot access our fat, we must look to alternate sources. Muscle is where our body turns, and slowly we eat away at our lean body tissue mass. Inside the muscle are mitochondria, the fat burning units, which are subsequently lost, thereby decreasing our potential to lose weight. In addition, it is the muscles that are responsible for supporting and protecting our joints.

For these reasons, it becomes clear that through a high carbohydrate diet it is almost impossible to lose weight while remaining in this bio-chemically undesirable state. Rising blood sugar levels stimulate the release of insulin, which ultimately stores the food we eat as fat. This is the process that has contributed to our society's weight problem; this is the effect we must reverse through our diet.

If we had maintained a balanced diet from childhood, we would not be trapped in the current nutritional crisis. Our bodies would not have developed insulin resistance and its attendant problems. Our goal is to retrain our bodies to a biochemical state similar to that of childhood. Once this is achieved, we can again enjoy a variety of different foods without gaining weight. To sustain this renewed metabolism and not undo or reverse the changes, balanced meals are still recommended.

The "naturopathic" diet is not a change in eating habits that we make temporarily until we lose weight and then return to the bad eating habits we had before. Any diet change that is not a lifestyle change only results in temporary weight loss. There is no need to restrict ourselves completely from all the foods we love, though. By making a few additions to our diet (instead of restrictions), we will be able to eat almost anything we wish after we have lost the weight. We can return to a large variety of different foods without any fear of regaining the weight.

Stage One: Weight Loss

The naturopathic diet progresses in two main stages. The first stage is the weight loss stage, lasting about 8 weeks. The diet here is protein-balanced and slightly carbohydrate restricted, especially complex carbohydrates. The second stage is the maintenance stage. Part of the maintenance diet is the addition of protein at each meal, but here the dietary choices expand, allowing us freedom to enjoy many different types of food. Weight loss ends but no weight is gained. If we return to a diet of high carbohydrates and low protein, though, we will undo all the metabolic changes that were brought about by the naturopathic diet.

For the first 8 weeks of this diet, we need to eat 15 to 25 grams of protein per meal. This size is approximately equivalent to the size of our hand. We may exceed this amount slightly but not go under it. We require this much protein to instruct the body not to secrete insulin at a high rate.

Common protein sources are listed below. There must be one protein source from the list below at every single meal. Although there are other foods that contain protein, such as lentils or yogurt, they are not high enough in protein to be considered a protein source. Drink as much water as possible because the protein forces your body to pass more urine

Protein Sources
Fish
Chicken/Turkey
Red Meat
Tofu (extra firm, low fat)
Eggs (3 egg whites to 1 yolk)
Protein Powders (use a whey protein powder, as it will also stimulate
    the immune system, with at least 15 grams of protein and only
    3 or 4 grams of carbohydrate)
Protein Bars (use bars that are high in protein but low in carbohydrates
    and fat; two-thirds of a bar is all that is needed for the protein
    portion of a meal and the rest may be snacked on later)
Low-fat Cottage or Ricotta Cheese (approximately 3/4 cup)

Legumes, such as lentils and chickpeas, must be considered a carbo-hydrate because they are approximately 70% carbohydrate and 30% protein, so try to limit their use.

Restricted Carbohydrates

High-sugar carbohydrates need to be cut, including all breads or bread type products, such as bagels and muffins, all pasta, rice, bananas, pota-toes, squash, corn, popcorn, yogurt, alcohol, and candy. This includes bread made with a grain flour other than wheat or rye, such as spelt and kamut flour, though a soy flour called "Dr Atkins Bake Mix" can be used as a substitute. This flour has no carbohydrate and is high in protein and makes very nice pancakes and muffins.

Limited Foods

Fruits need to be limited to a maximum of 2 pieces a day. Fruit is high in sugar and will force the body to secrete higher levels of insulin as well. It is important to note that one serving of fruit juice is equal to 1 piece of fruit.

All dressings, mayonnaise, butter, nuts, and cheeses are allowed but try not to use more than needed, for example, 1 slice of cheese and 5 nuts every other day. Do not replace the carbohydrates with fat.

You may have unlimited vegetables and salad including carrots, beets, and peas, but those that are high in carbohydrate, such as potatoes and squash, remain restricted.

Stage One Summary:

✦ 15-25 grams of protein per meal.
✦ Unlimited salads and most vegetables.
✦ Maximum of 2 pieces of fruit a day. No bananas.
✦ No grains, rice, pastas or starches.
✦ Very limited high carbohydrate, low protein foods
(e.g. chickpeas, lentils)
✦ Watch portion used of dressings or condiments.
✦ No alcohol.
✦ Keep up fluid levels by drinking water.

Stage Two: Weight Maintenance

The maintenance stage of the naturopathic diet is a true lifestyle pattern that we can easily maintain for the rest of our life. Throughout this second stage, our energy levels will remain high, our weight stable. We can enjoy every food group and continue to protect ourselves against many food related diseases at the same time. These benefits will last forever as long as we balance our protein and newly introduced carbohydrates at each meal. The maintenance stage is thus not so much a stage as it is a permanent change.

During stage two we begin to reintroduce the some of the carbohydrates that were eliminated or markedly reduced in stage one. Now that our body has consolidated the protein/low glucose message, it is possible to add in carbohydrates at a higher concentration, along with the protein, without increasing insulin release. Blood sugar levels will not rise rapidly as they did before, the reason being that the protein we are combining with the carbohydrates will slow the delivery of the sugar into the blood. This in itself will reduce the amount of insulin released. In addition, the reversal of insulin resistance and hyperinsulinemia achieved by stage one will further reduce the insulin response. Overall, less insulin will be secreted than before we started the diet. This will inhibit weight gain. Slightly more insulin will be released during stage two than during stage one, and this will prevent further weight loss.

When we reintroduce the carbohydrates, we will stop losing weight. We will not regain the weight we have lost, but the stage one weight loss process will stop. We may never ingest carbohydrates at the rate we did before or we may wish to incorporate them at every meal. The choice is ours.

The order in which we reintroduce the carbohydrates is very important. We must slowly integrate them back into the diet in a particular pattern. The sequence of reintroduction is determined by the glycemic index and type of sugar found in each carbohydrate. Fructose, the sugar found in fruit, is the first to be introduced. Then glucose from whole grains and breads, followed by pasta and rice, then potatoes and squash, and finally candy and alcohol. Following this approach minimizes large jumps in blood sugar levels and allows for easy adaptation of the body to carbohydrates.

Reintroduction Order

Fruits
Whole Grains, Breads, Cereals

Pasta
Rice
Potatoes and Squash
Candy and Alcoholic Beverages

The amount of carbohydrate brought back into the diet is also very important. We should reintroduce a small amount of carbohydrate initially, approximately 3 parts protein to 1 part carbohydrate at each meal (for example, 21 grams protein with 7 grams carbohydrate). We should remain at this level of carbohydrate intake for 4 to 5 days. A typical meal would be half a slice of bread, a piece of chicken, and unlimited salad or vegetable.

During this time period, we need to watch for signs of hyperinsulemia. Our body will become symptomatic when we ingest too many carbohydrates at once. We will feel tired shortly after the meal as our blood sugar levels drop too low. Several hours later or perhaps the next day we may feel bloated as our kidneys are not releasing enough salt. These signs will let us know that the ratio of carbohydrate to protein was too high and therefore insulin was secreted at a higher rate.

If none of these signs appear following the amount of reintroduced carbohydrate, then we can increase the amount consumed again. This time we might consider a ratio of 2:1 protein to carbohydrate. Again we need to watch for signs and symptoms of hyperinsulinemia. If they do not appear, we a can continue to increase slowly the amount and type of carbohydrate until we have reached a one to one ratio. Should the symptoms of hyperinsulinemia appear earlier, we have discovered our limit of carbohydrate intake and must return to the proportion previously used where no symptoms occurred. While a final fixed ratio of protein to carbohydrate cannot be quoted because it differs from individual to individual, as a general rule, a ratio of one part protein to one part carbohydrate, excluding vegetables and salads, is a fairly good balance.

This is our state of dietary balance. This is the ratio of protein to carbohydrate that we can ingest without changing our weight ever. At this balance between protein and carbohydrate, our blood sugar levels will remain steady and subsequently so will our insulin secretion and weight.

> ## Stage Two Summary:
>
> ✦ Continue 15-25 grams protein per meal.
> ✦ Continue unlimited salad/vegetable.
> ✦ Carbohydrate reintroduction:
> 1. Type - follow reintroduction order listed above
> 2. Amount - slowly reintroduce carbohydrates starting at a ratio of 3 protein : 1 carbohydrate
> 3. Increase - slowly increase the proportion of carbohydrate to protein towards 1:1
> 4. Watch for symptoms of hyperinsulinemia - If symptoms appear return to previous ratio at which no symptoms occurred
> THIS is your own personal protein solution!

By following this simple weight loss regime, the amount of force and pressure placed upon joints and the subsequent wear and tear within those joints will greatly decrease. By maintaining a normal healthy body weight and muscle mass, the support and strength surrounding each joint improves. When the muscles that bind to a joint are strong, that joint is better able to withstand the many forces and stresses placed upon it. In addition, the joint will rely more upon the muscle strength and less upon tendons, ligaments, and other joint structures for support. Once again, this helps to preserve the joint and decrease the progression of arthritis.

For more information on this diet, consult *The New Naturopathic Diet*, by Penny Kendall-Reed, with Stephen Reed.

Animal Proteins

There are some studies that show an improvement in arthritic symptoms when a diet low in animal products is used. Animal products increase the production of the chemicals responsible for inflammation in arthritis (prostaglandins and leukotrienes). Individuals notice that by removing the majority of animal products, especially red meat, from their diet, the symptoms associated with their osteoarthritis improve. After about 6 months, the body's sensitivity to these products falls, and symptoms only return 4 to 6 weeks after their reintroduction.

Some people may be particularly sensitive to certain types of animal products. To determine this, it is best to use a rotating diet. For 2 weeks, all animal products are removed. This includes all dairy products, chicken, turkey, red meat, pork, lamb, and eggs. By removing all the possible prostaglandin producing foods from the diet, the body will begin to clear itself of these excess inflammatory products and restore balance in favor of prostaglandins that decrease inflammation.

To determine which, if any, animal products you are sensitive to, eliminate all animal products, then choose one food type at a time and re-introduce it back into the diet every day for one week. Only bring one food in at a time in order to discover whether or not you are sensitive to that food. For example, bring in chicken, and only chicken, each day for one week. If no symptoms are present, such as increased pain or inflammation, keep the chicken in the diet and begin the same process with another food. If animal products have not been eaten for 4 to 6 months, it may take longer for symptoms to reappear. Continue with each food until all the foods have been tried. If at any point, an increase in pain is noticed upon reintroduction of a food, then remove that food at once. Wait 2 to 3 days before moving on to the next food so that the body has time to decrease its inflammation caused by the prior food type.

What most people discover is that there may be 1 or 2 foods within the animal food group that cause their arthritis to flare but they are fine consuming all others. Certain individuals may find that they remain asymptomatic as long as they moderate the amount of animal products they consume. For example, they may have no arthritic flares if they keep their animal product consumption to three times a week, but if they increase it to 5 times a week, their symptoms begin to return.

If all animal products are permanently removed from the diet, certain vital nutrients must be replaced. Vitamin B12 is a vitamin that is only found in animal products. It is important for the production of hormones, nerve transmission, regulation of certain cardiac factors like homocysteine, and it aids in the breakdown of fat and absorption of different nutrients. Similarly, much of our dietary calcium comes from animal products, such as milk, yogurt, and cheese. Calcium is crucial for proper bone metabolism. Without it, our bones are very likely to lose their density, adding to the risk of osteoporosis (loss of bone mineralization). Many of our iron sources are also from animal products. Although there are several vegetarian sources of iron, such as spinach and apricots, they tend not to be high in content, nor bioavailiable (readily absorbed and used by the body).

If animal protein is eliminated from the diet, it becomes very important to supplement these nutrients in the appropriate doses. A good general dose for vitamin B12 is 100-250 mcg a day with food. A healthy dose of calcium is 1200 mg a day, combined with 750 mg of magnesium for proper absorption and mineral balance. Finally, an appropriate dose of iron supplementation is 100 mg a day with food. Of course, all of these doses will vary slightly depending on the size, sex, age, and amount of exercise performed by each individual.

Nightshades

Other food considerations in treating arthritis are the nightshade or solanacea group of foods. These foods include tomatoes, potatoes, eggplant, peppers, and tobacco, which are quite alkaloid in nature. It is thought that the alkaloids inhibit normal collagen repair in the joints and actually promote the degenerative inflammation within the joint itself. Despite the fact that there is no significant clinical data to support this theory, some patients have reported great relief of arthritic symptoms through the removal of these foods from their diet.

Fasting

Although many of the same dietary principals apply to osteoarthritis and rheumatoid arthritis, such as weight loss and essential fatty acid supplementation, there are some aspects that are specific to rheumatoid arthritis. The concept that nutritional factors could alter immune and inflammatory responses has been studied extensively in rheumatoid arthritis. Initial investigation looked at fasting. Although there is no clearly established role for fasting in the reduction of arthritic symptoms, independent of the type of arthritis, there has been some data to suggest it may have a small role. One such study followed 15 patients with rheumatoid arthritis thorough a 7 to 10-day fast. Ten control patients were also examined over the same time frame. Five of the 15 patients reported a decrease in pain and stiffness compared to only 1 in 10 in the control group. However, long term fasting with a lacto-vegetarian low-calorie diet did not significantly improve symptoms further. This small study is by no means conclusive but suggests that short-term fasting may induce improvement in the symptoms of rheumatoid arthritis, but long term fasting is not necessary. The theory behind this is that by fasting there is a decrease in the permeability of the gastro-intestinal tract, reducing the absorption of protein allergens or inflammatory molecules, both of which have been suggested as affecting the disease process. The resulting reduction in inflammatory chemicals has been demonstrated.

Food Allergies

Allergies or sensitivities to food have also been considered in the development and progression of rheumatoid arthritis. Once again several studies have been published but there is currently no conclusive data, only possible theories. Food proteins can cause much the same reaction as a grass, mould, pollen, or any other allergen (peanuts, for example). When they enter the body in sensitive individuals, they evoke an immune response, releasing inflammatory mediators and causing hypersensitivity reactions. When food passes into the gastro-intestinal tract and acts as an allergen, the immune system produces an antibody that binds to the food in an attempt to neutralize it. This is known as an immune complex. One specific immunoglobulin that should help with the regulation and neutralization of these food allergens is IgA. However, it has been shown that the production of IgA is lower in individuals with rheumatoid arthritis than in unaffected people or those with non-inflammatory arthritis. It has also been shown that patients with rheumatoid arthritis have abnormal digestion and absorption of wheat and dairy products. Their gastro-intestinal tracts appear to be more permeable to these foods, making them acts as antigens or allergens.

Once again these results demonstrate that there may be a role for the specific detection and removal of allergens from the diet. Food allergy testing can be performed, but, in order to determine which food or foods that one is truly allergic to, it is important to perform valid allergy testing that examines the production of IgE and IgA in the blood.

NATURAL SUPPLEMENTATION TREATMENTS FOR ARTHRITIS

(5)

Nutritional supplementation is the addition of vitamins, minerals, and herbs to the diet for preventative and therapeutic purposes. This philosophy of supplementation has gained more acceptance over the past few years as we have become more aware of the deficiencies in our food. Not only are our 'fast-food' food choices lacking in vitamins and minerals, even our supposedly fresh vegetables and fruit are nutrient depleted. Our farm soils are exhausted, no longer enriched with natural minerals. Supposedly fresh foods have usually spent many days in storage or transport before making it to our plates. Food storage and processing generally destroys over 50% of the vitamin/mineral content in that food, though variations exist between different nutrients within the food. Baking obliterates 100% of vitamin B1, while processing damages 80% of vitamin B2. Given our over-processed, stale, nutrient-scarce diets, it is easy to see why nutrient supplementation has grown in popularity.

Vitamins are defined as any constituents in the diet other than protein, fat, carbohydrate, and inorganic salts that are necessary for normal growth and activity of the body. They must be obtained from external sources, and a deficiency may result in specific diseases, depending on the vitamin.

Minerals are essentially any inorganic substance found in the earth. Like vitamins, minerals must be taken in from an outside source and are necessary for proper bodily maintenance and growth. Minerals can be divided into two categories. *Macrominerals* are those that the body needs in larger doses of milligrams or even grams. These include such minerals as calcium, magnesium, phosphorus, and potassium. *Trace minerals* are those that are required in much smaller amounts, in micrograms. This category includes iodine, selenium, and chromium, for example.

Vitamins and minerals are essential components of enzymes and coenzymes. Enzymes are substances that stimulate different biochemical reactions in the body. Coenzymes aid the enzymes in this function. With proper nutritional supplementation, we can support certain enzymatic pathways to perform optimally, thereby speeding up certain reactions. If an enzyme is lacking a vitamin or mineral, it cannot function optimally and the process is slowed or halted. We must therefore ensure adequate nutrient supplementation to accentuate certain bodily functions.

Herbal supplementation is the use of botanicals or natural plants as therapeutic agents. Over 70% of prescription drugs are based on plant formulas. It follows that by using the original plant we can achieve a similar result. Botanicals or herbs will often have the same physiologic effect as a drug. They will bind to the same receptors and produce similar outcomes. The difference lies in strength. Generally, herbal medicine is much weaker, ranging from 1/100th to 1/1000th the strength of its pharmaceutical equivalent. Thus the natural medications require more time to have an effect. However, the benefit is that their side effects are generally minimal. Once again, by combining both forms of therapy, we can achieve a maximal effect with minimal side effects. This is done by decreasing the dose of pharmaceuticals and enhancing the therapeutic effect with natural supplementation.

The use of natural supplementation in the treatment of rheumatoid arthritis is not as established as it is for osteoarthritis. The variable presentation of the disease, its prominent inflammatory component, its systemic effects on numerous tissues and organs, and its potential for severe and rapid progression make traditional medical therapy essential in many instances. However, besides providing additional anti-inflammatory support and protection of articular cartilage, natural supplementation can help minimize the side effects of rheumatoid medication.

Selecting and Combining Supplements

Taking every supplement indicated for a particular condition is never advisable. It is best just to choose a few different natural substances that work in different ways and to then take the most effective dose of each. Many people have the philosophy that more is better, and the greater the intake of supplements the greater the benefit. However, what usually happens is that people sacrifice a sufficient dose of one supplement in order to take several others. Then the dose of each supplement ingested becomes too small to have a proper therapeutic effect. It is also important to avoid the situation whereby the taking of multiple supplements becomes so cumbersome that doses are missed or forgotten. These are all reasons why it is better to choose only a few specific products.

Although there are several very beneficial natural compounds available for the treatment of arthritis, it is important to choose one that is easy to take and will offer more than just pain relief. A wise choice would be one that has proven efficacy in treating the symptoms of arthritis, minimal side effects, and offers potential protection against further arthritic damage in the future. In our opinion, the supplements that best fit this picture are glucosamine sulfate, chondroitin sulfate, MSM, ginger, devil's claw, and curcumin. Not only are these among the most studied natural supplements, but they also have the greatest impact on pain, swelling, and other symptoms from arthritic joints. These supplements not only offer relief in terms of anti-inflammatory effects, but also appear to help repair damage already done and to prevent further damage upon a joint. They are available in many formulations, doses, and preparations.

Not all supplements will work equally well for everyone. We have found these natural remedies to be the most widely successful. However, if you do not achieve adequate relief, others can be tried from the following catalog of remedies. Just ensure you give them a chance to work, and do not change products too often. Natural supplementation for arthritis usually takes 10 to 14 days before any significant effect is noted. It should not be compared to the rapid onset of action of an analgesic or NSAID.

It is also important to recognize that your arthritis may need more aggressive treatment, such as pharmaceutical medicine, injection therapy, or surgery. Natural supplementation is just one weapon in a whole armory designed to help you beat your arthritis.

Supplement Quality

Few of the nutritional companies that offer products to consumers have the financial resources and infrastructure to guarantee absolute purity of raw material supply. It is not uncommon to find heavy metals, pesticide residue, and toxic micro-contaminates in products that consumers purchase. Our research has consistently led us to Jamieson Laboratories as one of only a few manufacturers in the world that integrates clinical protocols to guarantee the pharmaceutical purity of their raw material supply. Other suppliers felt to be reliable with respect to product quality include Quest, AOR, Sisu, Natura Pharm, Organika, and Natural Factors. Many of these products are available at regular retail pharmacies, health food stores, and specialty natural supplement outlets. Remember, if the product you are looking for is not available, most pharmacies will special-order it for you.

Glucosamine Sulfate

Glucosamine sulfate is the most widely researched natural therapeutic supplement used in the treatment of osteoarthritis. It is one of the primary building materials of cartilage and a vital component of the synovial fluid that lubricates a joint. Glucosamine sulfate is naturally produced by the body, but may also be taken in supplement form with a maximal absorption reaching approximately 90%. It has been used since the 1800s when it was isolated from chitin, a component in the exoskeleton of crustaceans, insects, and spiders.

Structurally, glucosamine is a molecule composed of glucose and an amine. The body uses this compound to make substances known as glycosaminoglycans or GAGs. The most important GAG with respect to joints is hyaluronic acid (HA). HA forms an essential part of the matrix 'glue' that binds articular joint cartilage together, attracting water and giving it structural properties to withstand the forces of joint impact and motion. It is also a critical component of the lubricating synovial joint fluid. HA winds like a snake between the collagen fibers that give the cartilage its strength. Other molecules called proteoglycans branch off from the side to increase its volume and ability to hold water. Chondroitin sulphate is an important component of these branches. HA and the proteoglycans not only hold water, they attract the minerals, vitamins, and other nutrients that maintain the integrity of cartilage.

As we age, we lose the ability to synthesize sufficient levels of HA, and the HA that is manufactured is smaller in size and subsequently less structurally effective. This results in a loss of strength, resilience, flexibility, and shock absorption within the joint. Glucosamine has been shown to slow this process down and help to repair and rebuild cartilage. It is for this reason that it is known as a chondroprotective agent. Not only does it reduce the symptoms of arthritis, but it appears to slow its progression.

There has been a great deal of research performed on glucosamine sulfate, confirming its use as a proven therapeutic agent in the treatment of oseoarthritis. In the laboratory, glucosamine sulfate has been shown to stimulate cartilage cells to synthesize GAGs, HA, and proteoglycans, the building blocks of cartilage. In another study, human cartilage cells from arthritic cartilage were put into culture and glucosmine sulfate added. The glucosamine sulfate increased the synthesis of proteins and protein kinase, promoting repair. It was also shown to decrease the activity of phospholipase A2 and collagenase, enzymes responsible for joint damage and cartilage breakdown. In simple terms, glucosamine sulfate, when added to these cartilage cells, promoted growth, repair, and cartilage synthesis – and inhibited further breakdown.

Clinical trials on the efficacy of glucosamine in the treatment of arthritis are abundant. Double blind trials in Portugal by 252 medical doctors on 1208 patients with osteoarthritis in the knee showed very positive outcomes where glucosamine sulfate was concerned. The patients were given either 1500 mg a day of glucosamine sulfate or a placebo for 3 years. The symptoms that were followed were pain at rest, pain on standing, and pain during exercise. Of the of the patients who were given the glucosamine sulfate, 59% reported significant decrease in pain in all three areas. This relief of pain lasted for up to 12 weeks following completion of the study and cessation of glucosamine sulfate.

Other studies have been performed comparing the use of glucosamine sulfate to ibuprofen for pain relief. A double-blind study consisting of 40 patients with osteoarthritis in the knee was performed over an 8-week period. Half of the patients were given 1500 mg of glucosamine sulfate a day. The other half were given 1200 mg of ibuprofen a day. Pain scores were then monitored over the entire 8 weeks. Results indicated that during the first 2 weeks, the group taking ibuprofen reported a more significant decrease in pain. However, by the end of the 8 weeks, the group taking the glucosamine sulfate had a much greater reduction in pain. Of great importance was that the group taking the glucosamine sulfate had a much better tolerance to their medications.

Similar studies compared the use of glucosamine sulfate with ibuprofen for temporomandibular joint osteoarthritis: 40 women and 5 men received either 1500 mg of glusoamine a day or 1200 mg of ibuprofen a day. Both groups had their doses split into 3, taking one dose 3 times a day. The study took place over a 90-day period. At the end of the study, 71% of the patients taking glucosamine sulfate significantly improved, compared to 61% of the patients on ibuprofen. Improvement was indicated by at least a 20% reduction in pain on function.

A review of 16 randomized, controlled clinical trials from the literature found evidence to support the effectiveness and safety of glucosamine sulfate in all 16. In 13 trials where glucosamine was compared to a placebo, it was more effective in 12. In 2 trials, it was more effective than an NSAID (anti-inflammatory medicine), and in 2 was equally effective.

All of the above studies are relatively short-term reports. Glucosamine sulfate has also been shown to have a potentially beneficial long-term effect on the progression of osteoarthritis. A study in the *Lancet* reported the effects of glucosamine sulfate on the knee over a 3-year period. A double blind randomized placebo controlled study was performed on 212 patients with osteoarthritis in the knee. They received either 1500 mg of glucosamine sulfate a day or a placebo. At the beginning of the study, specific examinations were performed. Weight-bearing, anteroposterior radiographs of each knee in extension were taken upon enrolment. The same x-rays were then retaken at 1 year and at 3 years. The knee joint was then assessed by digital image and the minimal joint space width (narrowest point between the tibia and femur) was taken by visual inspection with a magnifying lens. Of the 106 placebo patients, every single one had displayed progressive narrowing after the 3 years. On average, they had a narrowed joint space of 0.31 mm. However, no significant joint space narrowing was observed in the 106 patients taking the glucosamine sulfate. On average, their joint spaces narrowed by 0.06 mm. Symptoms of pain and mobility were reported to have worsened in the placebo patients, whereas symptoms improved in those taking the glucosamine sulfate. This study indicates that glucosamine sulfate may be a disease-modifying agent, useful in both the treatment and prevention of osteoarthritis.

Dose: The usual recommended dose of glucosamine sulfate is 1500 mg per day. This total amount should be divided into 3 doses of 500 mg per day. Larger doses may be taken at once, but the risk of adverse side effects increases as the dose increases. To help prevent any adverse side effects, the glucosamine sulfate may be taken with food. However, when any substance is taken with a meal, the absorption decreases slightly. Pain relief usually begins anywhere from 2 to 4 weeks and reaches its maximal effect around 8 to 10 weeks.

Safety: There has been no toxicity level of glucosamine sulfate reported to date. It is a very safe supplement with minimal side effects. The only reported side effects have been slight gastric irritation and diarrhea. These can usually be avoided by taking the glucosamine sulfate with a small amount of food. As glucosamine sulfate is derived from shellfish, anyone with an allergy to this should avoid this product. However, there are many glucosamine sulfate supplements that are no longer derived from shellfish.

It has been suggested that glucosamine sulfate may induce insulin resistance and promote the development of diabetes and obesity when used long term. This theory was based on studies in which *intravenous* glucosamine was given to rats. The effect does not appear to apply to humans taking oral supplementation. Two long-term studies in humans using oral glucosamine have demonstrated blood sugar levels to remain normal or slightly lower than those of control subjects taking a placebo.

Chondroitin Sulfate

Chondroitin sulfate is another component of the matrix 'glue' that maintains the integrity of joint cartilage. Chondroitin sulfate is a glycosaminoglycan (GAG) composed of two different molecules. The first component is a substance called galactosamine, which is chemically similar to glucosamine sulfate, yet structurally differently. The second component is glucaronic acid.

In Europe, chondroitin sulfate is used as an injection directly into the joint. This procedure has been successful in the reduction of osteoarthritic symptoms. In North America, however, there are no such preparations available, so oral supplementation is used. Unlike glucosamine sulfate where the absorption is excellent, ranging from 90% to 95%, the absorption of chondroitin sulfate is limited. The oral absorption of chondroitin sulfate has been shown to lie between 8% and 13%. The difference in absorption between glucosamine sulfate and chondroitin sulfate is due to the size of the molecules. Chondroitin sulfate is simply too large to pass through the normal gastro-intestinal wall. This has been demonstrated in studies, which show that following oral administration, blood levels of chondroitin sulfate did not change significantly. The size of chondroitin sulfate can be up to 300 times that of glucosamine sulfate. If by chance a smaller molecule of chondroitin sulfate did pass through, it would still be too large to be delivered to the chondrocytes (cartilage cells).

Clinical studies, however, do demonstrate clinical benefit, with reduction of symptoms, following administration of oral chondroitin sulfate. These results are supported in a number of other studies. In one such double-blind, placebo-controlled study, 85 patients with osteoarthritis in the knee consumed 400 mg of chondroitin sulfate twice a day, or a placebo. Pain on motion was the main symptom that was examined, but the physician's overall impression was also considered. A more objective symptom was calculated, too – the time required for each patient to walk 22 yards was reported. After only one month of treatment, there was a 23% reduction in pain reported by those patients taking the chondroitin sulfate as compared to only a 12% reduction in the placebo patients. At the end of the 6 months, 43% of the chondroitin sulfate patients reported significant improvement in pain, and only 3% of the placebo patients declared a similar reduction. Similarly, a small change was noted in the speed of walking between the two groups, whereby the patients taking chondroitin sulfate walked slightly faster and with more ease. The physicians overall impression was that chondroitin sulfate did appear to have a beneficial affect on osteoarthritic joints. There has also been radiological evidence for the benefits of chondroitin sulfate. Researchers found that in subjects taking chondroitin sulfate supplementation, joint damage in the knee, as followed by x-ray examination, did not progress over a one-year period. This was not found with those patients taking the placebo.

Thus it appears that chondroitin sulfate does have the ability to reduce pain and inflammation in osteoarthritic joints, as well as provide chondroprotective action.

But how does it work if it is too large to be absorbed into the chondrocytes? Chondroitin sulfate has been shown not only to stimulate cartilage repair mechanisms by offering partial building materials to the cartilage, but also to inhibit the enzymes that break down the cartilage. Other studies have shown an increase in hyaluronic acid following oral administration of chondroitin sulfate. A double-blind, placebo-controlled study reported in the *Journal of the American Medical Association* showed that patients taking supplementation of glucosamine and chondroitin sulfate had more beneficial effects for up to 3 years without any adverse side effects than glucosmine alone.

Dose: The recommended dosage is 400-500 mg, 2-3 times per day.

Safety: No adverse reactions have been reported with chondroitin sulfate. As with any supplement, food, or medication, the possibility of allergic reactions exists. If this occurs, stop taking it immediately and consult a physician. If any gastric irritation occurs, try taking smaller doses more frequently and with food.

Methylsulfonylmethane or MSM

Methylsulfonylmethane (or MSM, as it is more commonly called) is a naturally occurring sulfur-containing compound used in the treatment of arthritis. MSM contains approximately 34% elemental sulfur. It is a derivative of DMSO (dimethyl sulfoxide), another form of arthritis supplementation; however, when DMSO enters the body, only 15% of it is converted into MSM, the active molecule. MSM is found in many foods, such as fruit, alfalfa, corn, tomatoes, tea, and coffee. Interestingly, the richest source of MSM is in mother's milk. MSM is quite volatile and therefore its therapeutic effect is lost when food is cooked, processed, or stored.

Sulfur is needed to form connective tissue in the body and is essential for glycosaminoglycan (GAG) synthesis. It can be used to increase the production of s-adenosylmethione (SAM-e), glutathione, and N-acetyl cysteine. All of these substances individually influence joint and cartilage structure and function. GAGs are an integral part of articular cartilage structure. Sam-e and N-acetyl cysteine, as seen later in this section, contribute to the integrity of the cartilage matrix, attracting water and maintaining its shock-absorbing properties. Glutathione is one of the body's main free-radical scavengers, which decrease oxidation and inflammation. The role of oxygen free-radicals in the progression of arthritis is expanding, and glutathione acts to 'mop-up' these damaging molecules. Sulfur plays a crucial role in the maintenance of cartilage, and its concentration in arthritic cartilage is about one-third that of normal cartilage.

Our MSM intake is generally low as we eat insufficient whole, unprocessed foods where the MSM has not been broken down, making it particularly important to supplement with MSM, especially in arthritis.

Clinical studies thus far involving MSM are limited. One small investigation involved 16 patients with degenerative arthritis. Ten of these patients took 2250 mg of MSM per day and the remaining 6 had a placebo pill. Eight of the 10 patients taking the MSM reported a significant relief in 6 weeks with no adverse side effects.

Dosage: 750 mg to 1.5 mg per day.

Side Effects: The only side effect reported with MSM is a garlic odor on the breath.

Hyaluronic Acid

The most important GAG with respect to joints is hyaluronic acid (HA). HA forms an essential part of the matrix 'glue' that binds articular joint cartilage together, attracting water and giving it structural properties to withstand the forces of joint impact and motion. It is also a critical component of the lubricating synovial joint fluid. HA winds like a snake between the collagen fibers that give the cartilage its strength. In osteoarthritis, HA is found with decreased concentration and the molecules are smaller in size.

Injectable HA has been used for some time in both animals and humans and appears to have a beneficial effect in mild to moderate arthritis. Currently, most hyaluronic acid is administered through injection into the joint. It is theorized that an oral hyaluronic acid supplement may also stimulate cartilage to increase its synthesis of this essential molecule.

Dosage: 300 mg per day.

Side Effects: To date, there are no known side effects with oral supplementation of hyaluronic acid.

Ginger

For thousands of years, the ginger root has been used in Traditional Chinese Medicine to help decrease pain and inflammation. In recent years, research has demonstrated that the traditional use of ginger as a medication is both scientifically grounded and highly effective.

There are several different species of ginger. The most well known and most thoroughly studied is Zingiber officinale. Another well-documented species is Alpinia galanga, also known as greater galanga. This later species is the Siamese ginger plant. Both plants belong to the Zingiberacea family, which is comprised of well over 1300 different species. The rhizome (the underground stem, or root) is the medicinal part of ginger.

Pharmacologically, ginger root contains several hundred active ingredients. However, it is well recognized that the most important constituent of ginger is a group of substances known as the 4-hydroxy-3-methoxyphenyl (HMP) compounds. This group includes the active ingredients, gingerol and shogaol, both of which are types of oleoresins.

Ginger has many well-documented therapeutic uses, including anti-inflammatory and cholesterol-lowering properties. Several studies show that ginger is able to inhibit platelet aggregation by altering prostaglandin and thrombaxane synthesis.

Of greatest importance to the treatment of osteoarthritis is the anti-inflammatory effect that ginger has. Ginger operates in two different ways. When a tissue is injured, a group of immune modulators called cytokines are formed by the white blood cells. These cytokines, in particular inter-leukin-1 (IL-1) and tumor necrosis factor-alpha, give rise to the inflammatory process seen in arthritis. IL-1 and tumor necrosis factor can damage the articular cartilage of a joint and inhibit the function of cartilage cells. In addition, tumor necrosis factor and interleukin-1 stimulate production of enzymes that destroy or degrade the articular cartilage. The way in which ginger helps to combat this process is by preventing the white blood cells from liberating the cytokines at high rates. If there is less cytokine production, there will be less cartilage destruction and less inflammation and pain.

Ginger has another mode of anti-inflammatory activity. The balance of prostaglandins and leukotrienes in the body plays a very important role in the control of inflammation. There are various prostaglandins and leukotrienes that inhibit inflammation, while others promote it. Under normal circumstances, the body is able to monitor this balance and keep them in check. However, in arthritis, this balance is disturbed and there is an increase in the inflammatory prostaglandins, ultimately leading to the increased pain and swelling in the joints. There are two major enzymes that control the production of inflammatory prostaglandins and leukotrienes. These are cyclo-oxygenase 2 (COX-2) and 5-lipoxygenase. Ginger has an inhibitory effect on these enzymes, thereby decreasing the production of inflammatory prostaglandins and leukotrienes and subsequently their inflammatory effect on the body.

This is the same mechanism whereby the newest anti-inflammatories work. However, ginger does not appear to cause the frequent gastric irritation that the pharmaceutical anti-inflammatories do.

Clinical studies have demonstrated the effectiveness of ginger in the treatment of arthritis. One randomized, double-blind study of 261 patients showed significant improvement in knee pain for those taking ginger extract as compared to individuals taking a placebo. A cross-over study (in which patients are tested with the ginger and the placebo) by the same group confirmed these results.

Dose: 0.25 mg to 1 g, 3 times per day.

Side Effects: Occasional gastric irritation or dyspepsia has been reported in patients taking unencapsulated preparations.

Caution: Ginger may interfere with other medicines related to blood clotting. As with any medication, natural or otherwise, let your doctor know you are taking this supplement, and check before starting it if you are on any blood-thinning treatment. It should be stopped at least 2 weeks prior to any surgery.

Zinaxin

Another product we have found useful is a ginger extract, Zinaxin EV.EXT. In one double-blind, placebo-controlled study of patients with osteoarthritis in the knee, subjects took two Zinaxin capsules a day or a placebo pill. The study lasted for 6 weeks. Results showed that 2 out of 3 or 67% of those patients taking the Zinaxin reported a significant decrease in pain compared to the placebo group. A significant decrease in stiffness, increase in mobility, and decrease pain on walking was also reported.

Other studies conducted on Zinaxin have evaluated tissue samples from several patients with osteoarthritis. Zinaxin was found to reduce tumor necrosis factor and interleukin-1, both of which are chemicals responsible for inflammation and cartilage damage in arthritis. The results of the combined studies revealed that Zinaxin EV.EXT ginger extract had an equal or better effect than NSAIDs.

Dose: 250 mg, twice per day.

Side Effect: The only side effect experienced in some of the patients was mild heartburn or stomach irritation. The amount of irritation seen was much less than that of most pharmaceutical anti-inflamatories, including Aspirin and Tylenol.

Caution: See ginger above.

Devil's Claw

Devil's claw (Harpagophytum procumbens) is a plant indigenous to South Africa. A woody-barked plant that is claw like in structure, this plant produces bright red and purple flowers, but these appear to be devoid of any active ingredient. The root has long been used for digestive and rheumatological conditions. Its analgesic and anti-inflammatory properties are often compared to those of phenylbutazone.

In the United Kingdom, 30,000 people were reported to be using devil's claw for arthritic symptoms in 1976. Today in Europe, the European Scientific Commission of Phytotherapy has declared that this herb might be useful in the treatment of arthritis and tendonitis.

Devil's claw contains a number of active ingredients, such as iridod glycosides, phenolic acids, and flavinoids. The primary active ingredients, however, are the iridod glycosides, specifically harpagide, harpagoside, and procumbide.

Despite the popularity of this herb and clinical trials depicting its benefits, there still is no known mechanism of action. Many have suggested that it possesses the ability to alter prostaglandin synthesis, specifically that of eicosanoids. One such study involved 43 arthritic patients, each consuming 500 mg of devil's claw 3 times a day. After only 8 days, symptoms had improved. Patients reported an overall 89% reduction in pain, an 84% improvement in range of motion, and an 86% reduction in time needed for stiffness resolution. Other double blind placebo-controlled studies have been performed using this herb. In one such study, 50 patients with arthritis in various joints were monitored. These patients received either 800 mg of devil's claw 3 times per day or a placebo. At the end of the 8-week period, those patients taking the devil's claw displayed a statistically significant reduction in pain as compared to the placebo patients.

Although the way in which devil's claw works remains uncertain, the clinical evidence demonstrates that it may offer individuals a safe and effective form of treatment for their arthritic pain.

Dose: 500 to 1000 mg, 3 times per day.

Side Effects: Despite the fact that devil's claw has been compared to

NSAIDs, it does not appear to have the same gastric effects that other NSAIDs do. Occasional loss of appetite and headache have been reported.

Curcumin

Curcuma longa, otherwise known as turmeric, is a perennial herb that naturally grows in Southern Asia and throughout the Caribbean. It belongs to the ginger family and has traditionally been used primarily for flavor, especially in curry dishes. The useful parts of the plant are the rhizomes, or roots, from which volatile oils are extracted. Like boswellia, curcumin has been used in India for the treatment of inflammation and pain as well as an aid in the digestive process.

Curcumin's anti-inflammatory effects have been compared to hydrocortisone and phenylbutazone. Several different mechanisms have been shown whereby curcumin decreases inflammation in the body. The best documented is through the reduction of prostaglandin and leukotriene synthesis, achieved through the inhibition of, or interference with the enzymes that control the production of these inflammatory mediators (the 5-lipoxygenases).

Curcumin also acts in a variety of other ways. It has been hypothesized that curcumin inhibits the breakdown and metabolism of cortisone by the liver. This would increase the amount of circulating cortisone in the body and prolong its effect. Curcumin also appears less active in experimental animals without adrenal glands, indicating that the herb may also work by stimulating the release of adrenal corticosteroids. Further studies support a role for curcumin in the sensitization or priming of cortisone receptors. Cortisone is a powerful anti-inflammatory agent, and it might therefore be expected that these actions would increase its activity to reduce inflammation in arthritis.

Another mode of action that curcumin has been shown to posses is the inhibition of tumor necrosis factor (TNF) and interleukin-1 (IL-1). As seen in the section on ginger, tumor necrosis factor not only damages and breaks down the cartilage in the joints, but also increases the production of interleukin-1. Interleukin-1 increases the production and action of the enzymes that degrade cartilage. By decreasing the production of both of these cytokines, inflammation, pain, and joint damage will be reduced.

Clinical studies support the benefits of circumin in the treatment of arthritis. One study comparing the effects of curcumin to that of phenylbutazone (an NSAID) showed that patients improved equally, independent of which therapeutic supplement they were given. Arthritic patients in this study were given either 400 mg of curcumin, 3 times per day, or 300 mg of phenylbutazone, per day. Symptoms such as joint swelling, stiffness in the morning, and walking speed were monitored. Patients in both groups displayed equal relief and improvements in symptoms.

Dose: 400 mg of curcumin, 3 times per day. If you were taking the raw herb turmeric, this would equal approximately 7.5 grams per day.

Side Effects: Curcumin does not appear to have any adverse side effects. However, it may cause slight gastrointestinal upset with prolonged use. As turmeric has been shown to increase production and flow of bile, those with common bile duct blockage or gallstones should avoid this herb.

Capsicum

Capsicum is one of the most widely used spices in the world, with over 50 different species. We commonly see it in the red, yellow, and orange peppers as well as paprika, cayenne, and chili peppers. Capsicum gives a 'hot' sensation to food when used as a spice. As an herbal remedy, capsicum has been used in Mexico and Peru since around 7000 BC to increase circulation and aid digestion, but is now used primarily for its analgesic and anti-inflammatory properties.

The active ingredients in capsicum are the capsaicinoids, primarily capsaicin, which has a direct effect on inflammation and pain in the body. Shown to act through a specific receptor on pain fibers (the VR1 receptor), it decreases the production and action of substance-P. Substance-P is a chemical released from nerve fibers in response to pain. It mediates an inflammatory response by causing blood vessel dilation and the release of histamine from mast cells. At first, capsicum actually increases the release of substance-P. This can be seen in the burning sensation that is experienced after eating a hot pepper. However, with continued supplementation with capsaicin, substance-P production greatly decreases, reducing the overall pain/inflammation response. It was originally thought that capsaicin only affected those fibers that conduct the pain message from the skin to the central nervous system, but it is now thought that it has a wider effect on all sensory nerves and plays a central role in the spinal cord where substance-P acts as a neurotransmitter for pain stimuli.

Most forms of capsicum are administered through a cream and applied topically over the arthritic or painful area. The skin is supplied with many small nerve branches that then lead back to the main 'trunks' of the nerve. When capsaicin is applied to a nerve branch, substance-P is depleted simultaneously in all connecting branches, and hence it has its effect on the joint.

Several studies have been conducted on the efficacy of capsaicin, primarily in a topical cream form. One such study was conducted on 70 patients with osteoarthritis: 35 of these patients were instructed to apply 0.025% capsaicin cream a day, while the other 35 patients applied a placebo cream. After 2 weeks, 80% of subjects reported average pain reduction of 33%, significantly higher than the placebo group. In another study, topical capsaicin and glyceryl trinitrate were combined and compared to a placebo in a double-blind, randomized study. Pain scores and analgesic use were both significantly reduced in the treated group.

Dose: Creams generally range from 0.025% up to 0.075% of capsaicin. Due to skin sensitivity with these types of cream, it is wise to start with a lower concentration cream and slowly build up as needed. Remember, after the initial applications, the increase of substance-P will then reverse and that warm-to-burning sensation that may be experienced on the skin will deplete until it is no longer felt.

Side Effects: The main side effect experienced with capsaicin is a redness, irritation, and initial burning of the skin. These generally only last for a few minutes after application, and will subside with each following application until it is no longer experienced. *Do not use on damaged, inflamed, or broken skin.*

Boswellia

Boswellia serrata is a medium-sized branched tree that grows in the dry, mountainous regions of India. The purified compound obtained from this tree is a gummy resin known as guggul. This resin has been traditionally used in Ayurvedic medicine for treating chronic inflammatory states, such as ulcers and arthritis. During the last 10 to 15 years, some research has been performed on this compound to gain a better scientific understanding of its therapeutic properties. Boswellia appears to have anti-inflammatory effects in the body. It does not have any direct analgesic effect, but there is a significant reduction in pain through the decrease in inflammation.

The main active ingredients are the boswellic acids, predominantly salai guggul and olibanum. Their mechanism of action appears to be the reduction of leukotriene production without significant affect on prostaglandins. They work by interfering with the enzyme that controls the production of leukotrienes, 5-lipoxygenase.

This herb is used most widely in rheumatoid arthritis, but can also be a very valuable supplement in the treatment of osteoarthritis. Clinical studies have shown this herb to reduce in pain and swelling significantly. All forms of arthritis have similar inflammatory and pain characteristics, albeit to differing degrees. Boswellia appears to have a specific anti-inflammatory action, with success in rheumatoid arthritis and inflammatory bowel disease. It may prove useful in the treatment of all types of arthritis. Clinical investigation is ongoing.

Dose: The dose of boswellia is usually 350 mg to 400 mg, 3 times per day. If the patient is a young child with rheumatoid arthritis, then the dose may be cut in half. The extract is usually standardized to 38% boswellic acids.

Side Effects: Very few side effects have been reported with boswellia. There are rare reports of allergic reaction and nausea. Pregnant women are advised to avoid the intake of this herb until further studies have been performed.

Dimethyl Sulfoxide or DMSO

DMSO (dimethyl sulfoxide) is a bi-product of the wood industry, first introduced into the scientific world for therapeutic use in 1963. DMSO was extensively prescribed in Russia during the 1970s with up to 50% of Russian rheumatic patients taking DMSO as part of their therapeutic regime.

DMSO is now used widely all over the world without prescription for the treatment of musculoskeletal inflammation. Unlike MSM, DMSO is not found in the diet and must be taken in supplement form. When DMSO is ingested, approximately 15% of it is converted into MSM, one of its active components. DMSO therefore shares the healing and therapeutic qualities of MSM. It increases the moisture-retaining and shock-absorbing qualities of cartilage in a joint, increases free radical scavenging, thereby decreasing inflammation, and it provides building materials for collagen repair.

Besides its MSM-like action, DMSO has some primary effects with respect to arthritis. It acts as an anti-oxidant by neutralizing oxidized molecules in the body, particularly the joints. This decreases the number of free-radicals, molecules increasingly shown to influence arthritis and cartilage damage in arthritis. In clinical studies, oral DMSO has been shown to have significant effects on pain and inflammation in both osteoarthritis and rheumatoid arthritis. In one study, 318 rheumatoid patients used 90% DMSO liquid. There was a significant reduction in joint pain, improved range of motion, and increased grip strength.

The oral absorption of DMSO is excellent and its metabolism well established. It has also been shown to offer relief when applied topically, with effects lasting up to 6 hours. DMSO is most therapeutic when its concentration ranges from 70% to 90%. Anything higher and the efficacy actually starts to decrease. DMSO is administered in liquid, capsule, and topical cream form.

Dose: 1 quarter teaspoon of 90% solution in 8 oz water, taken daily.

Side Effects: Like MSM, the only known side effect is a garlic taste in the mouth and a garlic odor on the breath.

Willow

Willow or Salix has one of the longest histories of use in medicine, primarily for fever, gout, and inflammation. It has provided the foundation for many of the anti-inflammatory drugs used today. There are several species of willow, all of which belong to the family Salicaeae. The most common members of this family are crack willow or S. fragilis, black willow or S.

nigra, white willow or S. alba, and purple osier willow or S. purpurea. Despite the fact that the crack willow and the purple osier willow contain the highest concentration of active ingredient, the white and black willows are most commonly used in North America. It has been shown that crack willow and purple osier willow contain up to 10% and 8% active ingredient, respectively, whereas the white willow contains slightly less than 1%.

It is the bark of the willow that is used medicinally; bark of young branches is particularly rich in medicinal substances, particularly a glycoside known as salicin. However, salicin's anti-inflammatory effect is quite weak, requiring metabolism in the gastro-intestinal tract liver to reach its final form, salicylic acid (ASA or aspirin). This conversion takes time, so willow has a slower onset of action than salicylic acid itself, but the therapeutic effect of salicin appears to last longer than salicylic acid.

To speed up the onset of action of salicin and to increase its potency, a German chemist in 1835 created acetyl salicylic acid, aspirin, now one of the most regularly used anti-inflammatory, analgesic, and antipyretic (fever-reducing) medicines.

Dose: 20 mg to 40 mg of salicin, 3 times per day; or 1 2 ml of liquid extract, 3 times per day. This is equivalent to approximately 7-10 grams of dried herb, 3 times per day.

Side Effects: Despite the great success of salicylic acid, it does have adverse side effects. Salicylic acid is very irritating to the lining of the stomach where it can induce pain, nausea, and ulceration. In addition, salicylic acid decreases the blood's clotting ability by reducing platelet aggregation.

Salicin, however, does not appear to irritate the stomach. Very few people experience digestive upset or nausea with the use of willow alone. Salicin does have a mild effect on platelet aggregation, and use should be discussed with your doctor. Due to the mild inhibition of platelet aggregation, willow is not recommended in any one with a bleeding disorder, young children, pregnant women, or those with serious kidney diseases. In addition, willow can interact with other drugs, so it should be avoided in those people taking anti-coagulants, methotrexate, phenytoin, probenecid, spironolactone, and valproate. It should be stopped at least 2 weeks prior to any surgery.

SAM-e

SAM-e or S-adenosylmethionine is a substance formed by combining the essential amino acid methionine with adenosyl-triphosphate or ATP. ATP is the body's major form of energy storage. It is essentially three phosphate molecules attached together. When a bond between the three phosphates is broken, leaving a di-phosphate (two phosphates) and a single phosphate on its own, energy is released. This is the energy that our body uses to contract a muscle, conduct a nerve impulse, make the heart beat, or create an antibody. Our body uses ATP for every reaction in the body. It is this molecule that combines with an amino acid to form SAM-e.

SAM-e has been shown to increase the manufacture of certain cartilage components called proteoglycans. The blood levels of these proteoglycans rise following supplementation with SAM-e. Much as with glucosamine and chondroitin, SAM-e appears to have a beneficial effect on cartilage, and a potentially useful role in the treatment of arthritis. This role is mainly restorative, indirectly reducing inflammation by a reduction the destructive process. In one randomized, double-blind, placebo-controlled clinical study evaluating the efficacy of SAM-e, 734 osteoarthritic patients were evaluated over a four-week period: 235 patients received 1200 mg of SAM-e daily, 235 patients received a placebo, and the remaining participants took 750 mg of naproxen (a pharmaceutical anti-inflammatory). All of the involved patients were evaluated at the onset of the study, again at 2 weeks, and then at the end of the 4-week period. Symptoms that were followed were pain and ability to perform normal activities. Those patients taking SAM-e had as much pain relief as those taking the naproxen at the end of the study. Those patients taking naproxen did notice a decrease in pain much more quickly than those patients taking SAM-e; however, by the end of the study the pain relief between the two groups was equal. The naproxen treated group reported more side-effects, particularly stomach irritation.

An analysis of several clinical studies revealed that when patients consumed 1200 mg of SAM-e a day (400 mg, 3 times per day), there was a significant reduction in pain, stiffness, and other arthritic symptoms. The relief of symptoms achieved through SAM-e supplementation was comparable to that of several different NSAIDS, including ibuprofen, indomethacin, and piroxican.

SAM-e is very effective in the treatment of arthritis. Not only does it help to keep the joint healthy and strong by providing building materials to replace worn down cartilage, but it also helps indirectly to decrease the pain and inflammation of a joint through this repair.

Dose: 400 mg, 3 times per day. Once symptoms are decreased significantly, it is possible to maintain this beneficial effect at 200 mg, 3 times per day. It is best to decrease it to 300 mg, 3 times a day, for 1 month first. If the arthritic symptoms are still under control, then try a further reduction to 200 mg per day. Price is the main reason for the reduction in dose. It is a very expensive supplement.

Side Effects: SAM-e does not appear to have any adverse side effects, even long term. However, SAM-e does have anti-depressant properties and may actually elevate mood in those depressed due to chronic pain. If you are presently taking a pharmaceutical anti-depressant, it may interfere with the action and efficacy of the drug, so it is advised that you not take SAM-e.

Bromelain

Bromelain contains enzymes naturally found in pineapple. These enzymes have proteolytic properties, meaning that they help breakdown proteins into smaller units known as peptides. Other such enzymes include pepsin, trypsin, rennin, and chymotrypsin. Several beneficial results have been achieved by using these proteolytic enzymes as anti-inflammatories in such diseases as laryngitis, bronchitis, pneumonia, and also in sports injuries. Today, they are used extensively in the treatment of inflammatory joint disease, such as arthritis.

There are several ideas postulated as to the anti-inflammatory mechanism behind bromelain. The most popular postulates that it is mediated through the breakdown of fibrin. During inflammation, fibrin encourages the formation of matrix that walls or blocks off the inflamed area. This then leads to a build up of blood and edema around that area as it cannot be adequately drained. Bromelain promotes the degradation of fibrin, thereby allowing proper blood flow into the area and subsequent removal of inflammatory by-products that further injure the inflamed area.

It has also been shown that bromelain may block the production of the substances that are produced during an inflammatory reaction. These substances are known as kinins. By decreasing kinin production, there will be less swelling and inflammation and therefore less pain within the joint.

Studies have been performed to compare the use of oral enzymes in arthritis with that of traditional anti-inflammatories. One such randomized, single-blind study evaluated 50 patients with osteoarthritis in the knee over a 7-week period. Patients received either 2-3 enzyme tablets, 3 times per day, or 50 mg of the NSAID, diclofenac sodium. At the end of the study, a reduction in pain, joint tenderness, and joint swelling was seen in both groups. However, the reduction in pain was greater in those taking the enzymes ($p < 0.05$). A slight improvement in range of motion was also observed in the group taking enzyme therapy.

Dose: 150-300 mg per day.

Side Effects: Bromelain is a non-toxic substance that can be used in doses up to 1500 mg per day without fear of adverse effects. However, in some individuals, loose stools and mild blood thinning can occur. For this reason, those people already on blood-thinners should not take high doses of bromelain.

Arnica Homeopathic

Arnica is a natural anti-inflammatory and analgesic. As with all homeopathic treatments, the mechanism of action is unclear. Some studies indicate an effect significantly greater than placebo, while others have found no clear benefit.

Dose: 200 c (2 pellets), twice per day, dissolved under the tongue.

Copper

Copper is an essential trace element. Although it is only needed in small quantities by the body, copper plays a crucial role in many enzyme reactions.

Most of the copper in the body resides in the brain and liver, with lower concentrations in the muscles and bone. Copper can be found in oysters, shellfish, legumes, olive oil, walnuts, almonds, and other such foods.

Copper was first used by the ancient Greeks to relieve general aches and pains. Today, it is still used, although not quite as widely, for the same therapeutic reasons. Copper has been shown to have several modes of action for relieving pain. Copper may aid in the repair of collagen by increasing the action of the enzyme lysyl oxidase. By increasing the strength and integrity of collagen in articular cartilage, it may have a beneficial effect in arthritis. Copper also has anti-oxidant properties. Anti-oxidants neutralize free-radicals, molecules known to induce inflammation and accelerate cartilage deterioration. In contrast to other anti-oxidants, such as vitamins A, C, and E, copper does not act directly on the free radical, but rather increases the action of superoxide dismutase, one of the body's natural free radical scavengers.

The administration of copper via supposed skin absorption from a copper bracelet remains largely anecdotal; however, several studies have been shown a positive clinical effect in the treatment of arthritis. An open trial performed on rheumatoid patients showed positive effects. In this trial, most of the patients reported a decrease in pain and stiffness, but no mechanism for therapeutic benefit was offered. In another trial, patients wearing copper bracelets reported greater relief of symptoms than those wearing 'placebo' aluminum ones of identical design.

Dose: Generally, copper is administered though the topical application and absorption through the skin via a bracelet. If one were to take it orally, the dose would range from 1.5 mg to 3 mg per day. It should be noted that there are several different forms of copper, complexed with sulfate, picolinate, gluconate, or different amino acids. All have been shown to have equal efficacy.

Side Effects: Copper can induce nausea at doses of 10 mg per day, induce vomiting at doses around 60 mg per day, and is lethal at around 3.5 grams (3500 mg) per day.

Zinc

Zinc is a mineral used in every cell in the body. It is an essential co-factor in over 200 different enzyme reactions and aids in the production of several hormones. Zinc can be found in such foods as almonds, pumpkin seeds, ginger root, rye bread, oysters, and shell fish.

Zinc has been used, particularly in the treatment of rheumatoid arthritis, where serum levels are found to be low. Supplementation results in a slight decrease in pain and inflammation in these individuals. Zinc is also known to promote wound healing, to have an anti-inflammatory effect, and is essential for many immune mechanisms. Zinc is found abundantly in muscle, and plays an important role in its health and maintenance.

The beneficial effects of zinc are related primarily to its anti-oxidant properties, and as with copper, it helps to increase the function of the enzyme superoxide dismutase. By increasing the function of this enzyme, there is a subsequent decrease in free radical attack on cellular structures, and therefore a decrease in inflammation.

Although there appears to be a positive effect from zinc supplementation on arthritis, more studies should be performed to determine its efficacy adequately.

Dose: The usual range for zinc supplementation is between 30 to 60 mg per day for a therapeutic effect.

Side Effects: The main side effect that a chronic high dose supplementation of zinc would produce is a deficiency of copper. In doses of 2 grams per kilogram of body weight, consistent consumption can cause nausea and vomiting. Zinc can interfere with copper absorption and vice versa. Thus the dose of copper should be compared to that of zinc to ensure that there is not a depletion or inhibition of absorption of one or the other. In general, there should be 10 times more zinc than copper. For example, if the supplementation of zinc was 20 mg, then the supplementation of copper should be 2 mg.

Boron

Boron is another trace mineral that has recently received a great deal of attention with respect to bone and joint maintenance. Boron is essential to the structure of plants, but it was not shown to be crucial to humans until the early 1940s. We now know that boron is essential in the metabolism of both calcium and magnesium in the body, minerals which greatly contribute to bone health.

Boron can be found in almost all fruits and vegetables. This mineral is taken up from the soil into the plant. The boron content in the plant is dependant upon the boron concentration in the soil, and in general our soil contains sufficient levels to ensure acceptable levels in produce. It has been shown that the average American ingests 1.7 to 7 mg of boron per day. A diet rich in fruits and vegetables should be enough to ensure proper boron levels in the body.

Boron does appear to have an analgesic effect, although poorly investigated. In one double-blind, placebo-controlled trial, 20 patients with different types of arthritis were evaluated over an 8-week period. All the patients taking boron reported a decrease in pain and took less acetaminophen over the course of the 8 weeks. In the placebo group, only 1 patient reported this. Despite the significant results, no mechanism for analgesia was offered. Another study looked at the effects of boron on pain in osteoarthritis. Patients received 6 mg of boron per day: 71% reported a reduction in pain as compared to only 10% for the control group receiving the placebo.

Boron appears to play a role in the relief or reduction of pain in arthritis, but further studies should be performed to determine its exact mechanism.

Dose: 3-9 mg per day in general is a good safe dose.

Side Effects: Nausea and vomiting have been seen at doses higher than 500 mg per day. Boron has also been associated with increased estrogen levels. It is also possible that it may increase testosterone, but this is still under scrutiny. Once again, the mechanism by which boron may increase these hormones is not completely understood. If you are in a high-risk category for any hormonally related cancer, it is best not to use boron in supplement form.

Vitamin E

Vitamin E is a fat-soluble vitamin, whose main function is that of an anti-oxidant. Vitamin E is a constituent of every cell membrane, where it helps to stabilize the structure of the cell and protect it from free radicals. Vitamin E has a variety of other functions, including enhancement of the immune system. Of importance to arthritis is the role it plays in cartilage. Vitamin E appears to inhibit the breakdown of cartilage and stimulate the growth and production of new cartilage cells (chondrocytes).

Vitamin E is available in different forms, either natural or synthetic. The natural forms are d-alpha-tocopherols and the synthetic versions are the dl-alpha-tocopherols. It has been shown through several studies that the natural version has a greater absorption and biologic activity than the synthetic version.

Dose: The dose of vitamin E is approximately 400 IU per day. It can safely be increased to 800 IU per day (the usual dose for hot flashes). However, as an anti-oxidant, 400 IU is sufficient, particularly if it is combined with vitamin C as they have a synergistic effect together.

Side Effects: Because vitamin E is fat soluble, it can build up in the tissues if the dose is too high. This generally does not occur unless individuals are chronically taking more than 1600 IU per day. Vitamin E also has blood-thinning properties. It should not be combined with any other anti-coagulants, such as warfarin (coumadin), heparin, aspirin, or vitamin K. In addition, this vitamin should be stopped 10 to 14 days prior to any surgery. As with all medicines, let your doctor know if you are taking it.

Vitamin C

Vitamin C or ascorbic acid is a water-soluble vitamin. Vitamin C was first isolated in the late 1920s for the treatment of scurvy, and new roles for this important vitamin continue to be found. Vitamin C is an important free-radical scavenger in the body. Free radicals are known to mediate some of the damage and inflammation in arthritis. Blood levels of vitamin C are reduced below normal in patients with rheumatoid arthritis, and levels within joint fluid are even lower.

Although not extensively studied in the clinical setting, vitamin C does appear to have a potential role in the treatment of arthritis. The primary role is to help build and repair collagen. Vitamin C performs this function by increasing the binding together of amino acids to help support the structure of the collagen, an important structural component of cartilage. These amino acids specifically are proline and hydroxyproline. Vitamin C has also been shown to increase the production of proteoglycans, also structurally important molecules in cartilage. Several studies have been performed supporting this. One such study evaluated guinea pigs with osteoarthritis: cartilage erosion was decreased when the pigs were given high doses of vitamin C.

Dose: The dose for vitamin C is under continual dispute. Some experts, such as Linus Pauling, the Nobel Prize winner, recommend 2-9 grams per day, taking the vitamin until bowel tolerance (loose bowels) is reached. However, the recommended daily allowance for vitamin C is 60 mg. One end is too high and the other is too low. A good general dose is approximately 500 mg per day.

Side Effects: When vitamin C is taken in too high of a dose, loose stools or diarrhea results. Otherwise, there are no adverse reactions with vitamin C.

Essential Fatty Acids

Most people try to stay away from fatty foods, and for the most part, this is a wise decision. However, there are some fats that are actually beneficial – indeed, essential to the body. Most people are approximately 70% to 80% deficient in essential fatty acids. The symptoms of a low dietary intake of essential fats are fatigue, dry skin and hair, constipation, depression, bloating, and arthritis.

All fats, whether they are good or bad fats, have a similar basic structure, that is, a molecule of glycerol and three fatty acids. Fatty acids come in a variety of different shapes and sizes and they perform a multitude of different functions in the body. For instance, fats surround each cell in the body and act as a barrier, protecting the cell from metabolic toxins and allowing hormones and enzymes to bind to it. Fats are also an energy source for the body. The fats that are actually good for us are known as essential fatty acids. There are four main types of essential fatty acids, omega-3, omega-6, and omega-9 and 7. These are unsaturated fats, meaning they have one or more double bonds connecting their chemical structure. It is this double bond property that allows them to interact with other substances in the body.

Omega-3 Essential Fatty Acids

Omega 3 fats are broken down into three different groups. The first are alpha-linoleic acids. They are found in flax seeds, hemp seeds, canola, soy, walnuts, and dark green leaves. The second group are stearidonic acids and are found in blackcurrents. The final group, eicosapentaenoic acids, are found in cold-water fish like salmon, mackerel, sardines, and trout.

Omega-6 Essential Fatty Acids

Omega 6 fats are also broken down into three different groups. The first group is the linoleic acids or LAs, which are found in safflower, sunflower, hemp, soybean, pumpkin, and sesame. The second group, gamma-linolenic acids or GLAs, are found in borage oils, evening primrose oil, and blackcurrent seed oil. The final group of omega-6 fatty acids are the arachidonic acids found in meats and other animal products.

Omega-7/9 Essential Fatty Acids

Omega-9 fats are also called oleic acids and are widely abundant in olives, almonds, avocados, peanuts, cashews, and macadamia oils. Omega-7 is found in coconut and palm oils. These fatty acids do not play a crucial role in the treatment of osteoarthritis.

The relative ratio of these fats in the body is crucial in determining which prostaglandins will be produced. Prostaglandins are hormone-like substances and are important in the regulation of many bodily functions, such as blood pressure, pain, inflammation, swelling, allergic reactions, blood clotting, and more. Inflammation in arthritis is mediated by such chemicals as prostaglandins and leukotrienes. The body also produces 'good' prostaglandins that moderate inflammation and have other important protective functions. The role of essential fatty acids in the treatment of arthritis is to limit the availability of arachidonic acid, the base molecule from which prostaglandins are manufactured. They seem to promote the preferential manufacture of 'good' prostaglandins. While some fats, like those found in animal products, promote the synthesis of inflammatory ('bad') prostaglandins, the omega-3 and 6 fatty acids lead to the production of the more beneficial molecules.

The main goal of essential fatty acid supplementation is to decrease the production of arachidonic acid and increase the production of eicosapentaenoic (EPA) and dihomo-gamma-linoleic acids (DHGLA). These latter two are the final products of omega 3 fatty acids and omega 6 fatty acids, respectively. Several studies have been performed using essential fat supplementation and measuring the relative levels of EPA and DHGLA. For example, when a diet rich in omega 6 fatty acids was followed (1.5 tablespoons/day of flax oil), the levels of EPA rose significantly in the participating individuals.

Clinical evidence for the efficacy of essential fatty acids in the reduction of inflammation associated with arthritis is growing. In one crossover study, patients received either 2.7 grams of eicosapentanoic (EPA) or a placebo. A significant reduction in arthritic symptoms was observed with the EPA. In another study, significant reduction in inflammatory chemical (leukotriene) synthesis was seen.

Essential fatty acids can help to decrease the production of inflammatory mediators, thereby decreasing pain and inflammation in a joint. Essential fatty acids also help to improve the ratio of good to bad cholesterol, soften skin and hair, and regulate bowel movements. Due to all of these other beneficial side effects as well as the decreased inflammation, EFAs are a wise adjunct in the treatment of arthritis.

The important issue then becomes achieving the correct balance of different fats in the body in order to decrease osteoarthritic inflammation. The most favorable ratio of omega 6 to omega 3 essential fatty acids is approximately 4:1. However, it is important to note that most dressings and oils in the grocery store contain omega 6 oils. Thus many people are already consuming it in high quantities. In fact, many people are consuming a ratio of 15:1 of omega 6 to omega 3 fatty acids. The most viable solution is to increase the omega 3 fatty acids. This is easily achieved by consuming more flax seed oil, which has a relative ratio of 1:3 of omega 6 to omega 3 fatty acids.

In order to determine which fatty acid supplementation is best for you, it is important to consider all the different fats already in your diet. If you generally follow a very low fat diet, then you should consider a mixed essential fatty acid supplement that contains both omega 6 and 3, with a slightly higher concentration of omega 3 to counteract the hidden omega 6 fatty acids that will undoubtedly exist in your diet.

Dose: The dose of essential fatty acids that is of most benefit is approximately 4-5 g per day with food. The ratio in general should be around a 4:1 omega-6 to omega-3 fatty acids.

Safety: Essential fatty acids are very safe. There is no real toxicity level associated with essential fats. However, they can cause some gastro-intestinal changes, such as belching after consumption and loose stools when the dose is too high. If you already have loose stools, it is advisable to drop the dose in half.

Many essential fats come from cold water fish so it important to ensure that you are not allergic to these sources. Fish oil supplementation can have an effect on blood clotting. In high dose, it can slightly thin the blood and should therefore be used with caution if you are taking blood thinning medication, such as warfarin, heparin or high dose aspirin. If you are predisposed to easy bleeding and are on high doses of other vitamins that can contribute to thinning of the blood like vitamin E and C, then you should consult a health care practitioner to determine the correct dose for you before starting essential fatty acid supplementation.

Arthrimin

There are several products available that blend natural supplements. Arthrimin is well tolerated and has good clinical backing. Arthrimin GS, an effervescent powder, is a mixture of glucosamine sulfate, chondroitin sulfate, MSM, and hyaluronic acid. The doses of each are as follows:

Glucosamine Sulfate	1500 mg per package
Chondroitin Sulfate	1200 mg per package

MSM   1000 mg per package
Hyaluronic Acid   300 mg per package

As these substances have essentially no adverse side effects, it is possible to begin with a higher dose, reduce inflammation, initiate repair, and then decrease the dose as needed. An appropriate dose would be one package per day for 4 to 6 weeks, on an empty stomach, and then decrease to one package every other day.

A study using Arthrimin GS was performed on 46 patients with osteoarthritis. Over a 10-week period, patients took one package of Arthrimin GS a day on an empty stomach. Symptoms were evaluated using a visual analog scale at the beginning of the study and at the end of the 10 weeks. The symptoms followed were pain, stiffness, mobility, swelling, sleep, and overall health. Other natural supplements for arthritis were stopped prior to the study. The results are illustrated in the chart below. Statistical analysis indicated these results were highly significant.

Parameter	Percentage of Patients Showing Improvement	Average Percentage of Improvement
Pain	80.4 %	24 %
Stiffness	84.8 %	22 %
Mobility	76.1 %	16 %
Swelling	63.0 %	14 %
Sleep	60.9 %	10 %
Health	69.6 %	14%

Of the patients in the study, 8 were taking NSAIDs; 5 out of these 8 patients reported reducing their dose, and 3 of the 8 patients discontinued anti-inflammatories completely. Additionally, 5 patients participating in the study were taking advil/tylenol for their arthritic pain; 3 out of these 5 patients were able to stop taking their daily doses of these medications during the study due to the relief they found from the Arthrimin GS.

Subjects reported that the product was easy to take, the equivalent dose in pill form being 9 capsules per day. The powder formulation is thought to improve absorption of the component supplements.

Treatment of Side Effects

Besides providing additional anti-inflammatory support and protection of articular cartilage, natural supplementation can help minimize the side effects of regular arthritis medication. If you are taking an anti-arthritis drug, the supplements listed here may reduce side effects. It is important to discuss any new medication or supplement with your medical or naturopathic doctor, particularly if you taking a number of different therapies.

Slippery Elm, Marshmallow, and Cabbage

Slippery elm, marshmallow, and cabbage are all demulcent, emollient herbs that help to soothe irritated and inflamed mucous membranes, such as the bowel.

Dose: 350-500 mg of each, 3 times per day, without food.

Quercitin

Quercitin is a bioflavinoid, which acts as a natural anti-histamine by binding to the cell that produces histamine (mast cell), decreasing its production of histamine.

Dose: 600 mg, 2 to 3 times per day, without food.

Acidophilus (Lactobacillus acidophilus)

Acidophilus (Lactobacillus acidophilus) is the "good" bacteria that normally inhabits the bowel and helps to maintain the normal bacteria floral balance, prevents yeast and fungal infection, and helps to regulate bowel movements.

Dose: 1-3 capsules per day with 1 billion bacteria per cap on empty stomach.

Milk Thistle

This herb is a liver protective and liver detoxification herb that helps to protect and clean out the liver.

Dose: 500 mg, twice per day, on an empty stomach.

Lemon

Lemon directly stimulates the detoxification processes within the liver.

Dose: 1 tsp per day, in warm water, in the morning.

Globe Artichoke

This herb helps to break down uric acid crystals and helps both the gall bladder and liver clean and recycle products.

Dose: 250 mg, 3 times per day, on an empty stomach.

Zinc

This mineral is used to help stimulate cellular turnover and wound healing.

Dose: 25 mg per day, with or without food.

Vitamins A and E

These anti-oxidant vitamins reduce free radical damage and inflammation.

Dose: Vitamin A, 10 000 IU per day; Vitamin E, 200 IU per day.

5-HTP

5-HTP is a precursor to serotonin (our so-called 'happy hormone') and increases production of this hormone.

Dose: 50mg, twice per day. Should not be taken if you are on any other anti-depressant medication.

Kava Kava

A nervine herb, kava kava decreases the release and the effects of cortisone.
Dose: 200-300 mg, twice per day. Avoid in the presence of liver disease.

St. John's Wort

This anti-depressant herb increases the re-uptake of serotonin.

Dose: 350 mg, twice per day. Should not be taken if you are on any other anti-depressant medication. Increases skin sensitivity to sunlight.

Vitamins B-6 and B-12

These vitamins improve nerve transmission and stimulate the production of serotonin.

Dose: Vitamin B-6, 100 mg, twice per day; Vitamin B-12, 250 mcg, once per day. Both should be taken with food.

Calcium-Magnesium

These minerals are used to control muscle contraction and reduce spasm.

Dose: Calcium 500mg/Magnesium 350mg, twice per day.

Treatment Guidelines with Arthritis Medications

NSAID Side Effects

– Gastro-intestinal (GI): zinc, slippery elm, marshmallow, cabbage

Methotrexate Side Effects

– Mouth/GI : zinc, slippery elm, marshmallow, cabbage
– Low folate: vitamin B complex (folic acid)
– Liver toxicity: milk thistle, lemon

Prednisone Side Effects

– Weight gain, fluid retention, high cholesterol, high blood pressure:
      the naturopathic diet
– Osteoporosis: calcium, magnesium, zinc, hydroxyapatite

6 | MEDICATION TREATMENTS FOR ARTHRITIS

A dvances in pharmaceutical treatments for arthritis have been rapid over the past 10 years. Every month seems to bring a new 'wonder drug' with greater efficacy and fewer side effects. This section aims to offer information on these medicines and some guidelines as to their use. These descriptions do not constitute complete drug monographs. Contraindications and warnings should be read and discussed with your pharmacist or doctor before starting any new medication.

Painkillers (Analgesics)

Painkillers are the first line in the medicinal treatment of arthritis, although in the presence of acute, severe swelling and inflammation, particularly when this is associated with one of the more systemic inflammatory arthritis diseases, such as rheumatoid arthritis or gout, other medications will be necessary. For the early symptoms of arthritis, especially osteoarthritis, a simple analgesic such as ASA (acetylsalicylic acid, aspirin), tylenol, or acetaminophen is extremely useful. However, acetaminophen and ASA should be used only intermittently for pain. ASA has more anti-inflammatory action but is less well tolerated, particularly in older individuals. Neither drug should be used excessively on a long-term basis. Pain requiring such prolonged use likely needs an alternate medication.

Because of its more significant anti-inflammatory activity, ASA is likely more effective at reducing swelling and inflammation than acetamino-phen but has similar pain killing properties. Gastric side effects are more frequent, including indigestion, gastritis, ulcers, and bleeding. ASA also reduces the ability of the blood to form clots, increasing risk of bleeding. ASA should not be used in the presence of active stomach ulceration, and its use should be reconsidered with a prior history of this condition, especially if associated with bleeding. ASA treatment should be stopped 10 days prior to any surgery due to its effect on blood clotting, and should not be used in individuals with a history of clotting problems.

Acetaminophen has painkilling activity equal to ASA but does not have such anti-inflammatory activity. It is not associated with bleeding from the stomach and does not interfere with blood clotting, two of the possi-ble side effects of ASA. Excessive use of acetaminophen, however, can have significant effects, with possible damage to the liver, and can interfere with blood-thinning medicines.

Non-Steroidal Anti-Inflammatory Medications (NSAIDs)

Non-steroidal anti-inflammatory medications are a group of drugs that include ASA and act specifically to control inflammation. By blocking an enzyme involved in the production of inflammatory chemicals (prostaglandins), NSAIDs, like ASA, can have a dramatic effect on reducing and controlling inflammation. These beneficial effects are not without a risk to other areas of the body, however. The most significant of these is the possibility of causing ulceration and bleeding in the stomach. NSAIDs should not be used in patients with active ulceration or bleeding; a history of this condition in the past is a relative contraindication to their use. The risk increases with age over 60 and smoking. Older NSAIDs also affect blood clot-ting and should not be used with a history of bleeding disorder or at the same time as anti-coagulants. They should be stopped 10 days prior to surgery. NSAIDs should be avoided in patients with kidney disease or heart failure.

Recently, a new type of NSAID has been developed. These are the so-called COX-2 NSAIDs and include rofecoxib and celecoxib. The enzymes responsible for the production of chemicals mediating inflammation (prostaglandins, leukotrienes, etc) are the cyclo-oxygenase or COX enzymes. There are two types. The COX-2 enzyme is particularly involved in arthritis and inflammation, and has been shown to increase its activity greatly during acute episodes. The COX-1 enzyme, which is constantly present at certain levels in all tissues, appears to produce similar chemicals that are of value to the body and protect it, particularly in areas such as the stomach. The older anti-inflammatories did not distinguish between these two enzymes and side effects were therefore more frequent. The COX-2 NSAIDs have less stomach irritation and do not interfere with blood clotting.

Rofecoxib and celecoxib do have their own set of side effects, however. Celecoxib cannot be taken if you have an allergy to sulpha. They both affect the kidney and can cause fluid retention in susceptible individuals, which may cause an increase in blood pressure. There has been recent concern as to whether COX 2 medications increase the risk of heart attacks. Although the risk is slight, it appears primarily due to the fact that the COX-2 NSAIDs, unlike ASA and COX-1, do not have a blood thinning effect on the clotting cells or platelets. While this is beneficial in reducing bleeding episodes and making reversal easier for surgical procedures, it likely removes the protective effect on the heart. It has been suggested, therefore, that in susceptible individuals ASA treatment in low dose be continued along with the COX-2 NSAIDs.

Interestingly, with regards to efficacy in the treatment of osteoarthritis or rheumatoid arthritis, no one anti-inflammatory has proven to be superior to another, or indeed to ASA. However, there does seem to be a tremendous variability in tolerance to these medications and in how well they work between individuals.

Doctors will usually prescribe an NSAID they have administered before with success for patients in your situation. The prescribed medication should be tried for about 2 weeks. If at that stage it is not working or there are intolerable side effects, then it can be changed. Factors such as cost, pill size, frequency of medication, effectiveness, and side effects are all factors in choosing the right NSAID.

All NSAIDs are associated with rare side effects, such as skin rash, liver and kidney problems, asthma, dizziness, and headaches. The main side effect is indigestion or stomach ulceration and bleeding. About 1 in 100 patients who take anti-inflammatories for 1 year will develop an ulcer, and about half of those will get bleeding problems. Unfortunately, not all ulcers cause symptoms of heart burn or indigestion, and the first sign of trouble may be bleeding, causing black tar bowel movements, low blood count, dizziness, and fainting.

It is possible to prescribe a stomach protective agent as an additional medication. Some NSAID preparations actually include this. Problems, however, can still occur. The highest risk comes from continued use of anti-inflammatories. This may well be minimized by intermittent use. Arthritis pain is usually periodic in nature, with patients noting marked pain and swelling for a few weeks, after which the joint settles down. NSAIDs can be used quite effectively during these periods and then stopped once the joint settles down.

Use of a natural arthritis supplement may allow you to reduce the frequency or dose of NSAID and thus the potential side effects. See also "Treatment of Side Effects" in the preceding chapter on nutritional supplements.

Disease Modifying Anti-Rheumatic Drugs (DMARDs)

Medical management of rheumatoid arthritis remains the mainstay of treatment for this form of the disease. It becomes increasingly important as the severity of the disease progresses, not only to control the pain and swelling around joints, but to reduce the involvement of other areas, such as the eyes, lungs, and heart.

Initial treatment may involve the analgesics and NSAIDs noted above. However, the more acute and severe the presentation of the arthritis, and the more extensive the involvement of other tissues and organs, the more likely it is that the following drugs may be incorporated into management.

Failure of NSAIDs to give sufficient relief of symptoms is an indication to move to second-line drugs or DMARDs (disease modifying anti-rheumatic drugs). These include oral steroids, anti-malarials, sulfasalazine, gold compounds, penicillamine, methotrexate, and azathioprine. These powerful drugs reduce disease activity, although their mechanism of action is often unclear. They have significant side effects and numerous drug interactions.

Corticosteroids (Prednisone)

Corticosteroids are hormones produced by the adrenal gland in normal individuals. Cortisone is the so-called stress hormone essential for allowing the body to adapt to stressful situations. In response to stress, cortisone will produce increased blood sugar, increased alertness, increased muscle metabolism, and improve detoxification. As a drug, cortisone was isolated in the 1930s, but its impressive role as an anti-inflammatory agent was not discovered until the 1950s. Unfortunately, this panacea for inflammatory ills has proved to have many serious side effects, which have curtailed much of the initial enthusiasm for its widespread use. It remains, however, pivotal in the treatment of inflammatory arthritis.

Cortisone is generally given as oral prednisone therapy. Doses greater than 7.5 mg per day are associated with a greater incidence of side effects, although problems are relatively common even in lower doses. The drug is generally used for acute flare-ups of inflammation, and patients with rheumatoid arthritis are generally able to modify their dose to account for variations in their disease. Steroid injection into a joint can be a useful interventional therapy when one or more joints are involved in an acute flare-up of the disease.

Side Effects:
- hypertension
- osteoporosis
- osteonecrosis
- truncal obesity
- impaired wound healing
- acne
- high blood sugars
- high blood lipids and associated hardening of the arteries
- fluid retention
- increased infection risk
- muscle pain and weakness
- mood alterations including euphoria, insomnia, and depression

Anti-Malarial Drugs

The development of anti-malarial drugs for the treatment of rheumatoid and other inflammatory forms of arthritis arose from anecdotal reports and observations by British physicians. The mechanism of action by which the anti-malarial drugs act is not completely clear, but it appears related to changes in cell acidity that influences the production of chemicals that mediate the inflammatory process.

The most commonly used drugs are chloroquine and hydroxy-chloroquine, both of which are taken by mouth. They are probably most beneficial in the early stages of rheumatoid arthritis as they result in decreased joint inflammation, swelling, and stiffness. They are also shown to be particularly effective in children with juvenile rheumatoid arthritis.

The risks associated with anti-malarial use are considerably less than many of the other DMARDs, so long as the recommended dose range of 6 to 7 milligrams per kilogram per day is maintained. The drugs are also useful in SLE.

Side Effects: The most common side effect is gastric upset. The most serious involves damage to the retina in the eye, but in the recommended doses this is uncommon, and, if monitored closely, is reversible. Skin rashes occur in up to 5% of patients, and, in darker skinned patients, lightening of certain areas of the skin may occur.

Gold Compounds

Gold salts were used as far back as the 19th century for the treatment of infections, including tuberculosis. Early experience with the success of gold salts led to the idea that rheumatoid joint inflammation may be due to infection.

Gold salts are recognized as being effective in suppressing inflammatory activity in rheumatoid arthritis. The mechanism of action remains unclear. Treatment with gold salts results in improvement in joint symptoms and may slow progression of joint destruction. The levels of certain blood markers of rheumatoid arthritis have also been shown to be reduced.

Most gold preparations are given by injection, with the exception of auranofin, which can be taken by mouth.

Side Effects: About one-third of patients experience side effects, which include mouth ulcers, skin rashes, kidney damage, reduced production of blood cells by the bone marrow, diarrhea and colitis, lung inflammation, and damage to nerves causing numbness and tingling.

D-Penicillamine

Like gold, the specific action of D-penicillamine in the treatment of rheumatoid arthritis is not known. The drug has been shown to alter white cell function and may reduce the production of rheumatoid factors. D-penicillamine binds certain minerals in the blood, and this may reduce the activity of certain destructive enzymes, such as collaganase.

D-pencillimine is given by mouth initially at a small dose with the dose gradually increased. It needs to be taken on an empty stomach or else it will not be absorbed. The dose is gradually increased over about three months and it is not until this time that the patient begins to experience relief of symptoms.

In clinical trials, D-pencillimine has been shown to be as effective as gold and azothiaprine. Unlike gold, it has been shown to be more effective at improving symptoms of rheumatoid arthritis in areas other than the joints. However, D-penicillamine is now rarely used in the treatment of rheumatoid arthritis.

Contraindications: Despite its derivation from penicillin it is not contraindicated in patients with an allergy to penicillin.

Sides Effects: Side effects include mouth ulcers and skin rashes, kidney damage with protein reduced production of blood cells, and lung inflammation.

Methotrexate

Methotrexate is probably the most popular and routinely used DMARD in rheumatoid arthritis. Numerous clinical studies, a position paper from the American College of Physicians, and approval by the FDA in the mid 1980s have supported its efficacy. Methotrexate is also used in psoriatic arthritis and SLE.

Methotrexate is a potent drug that, in higher doses, is used in chemotherapy for such cancer conditions as choriocarcinoma and leukemia. At lower doses, it is a first line DMARD for rheumatoid and other forms of inflammatory arthritis. It acts by inhibiting enzymes involved in the metabolism of folic acid. It appears to interfere with the function of cells involved in the inflammatory process and decreases levels of such chemicals as interleukin-1 and leukotrienes. It may also have an immune suppressive effect to reduce the production of some auto-antibodies.

Methotrexate is given by mouth and in most patients is absorbed rapidly. Response occurs within a few weeks of treatment initiation with reduced inflammation, swelling, and stiffness, improved function, and slowed disease progression. Withdrawal of the drug often results in a flare-up of the disease within a few weeks.

The average weekly dose of methotrexate is about 12.5 mg, with a range of 5 mg to 50 mg. Treatment is usually initiated at a lower level and gradually increased.

Side Effects: Side effects of methotrexate vary greatly in severity. Their incidence increases with reduced kidney function, deficiency of folic acid, increased age, and use of other drugs. The most common side effects involve the mouth and gastrointestinal tract, where painful ulcerations can occur. These are effectively treated in the administration of folic acid. Reduced blood counts can occur and should be continuously monitored. In rare cases, this reduction can be severe. Damage to the liver does occur but is less frequent with current dosing regimes, about 1 per 1,000 patients over a 5-year period. Regular intake of alcohol is contraindicated. Inflammation of the lungs and cardiovascular system is rare and skin rashes usually mild and reversible. Other side effects include reduced wound healing and an increased risk of infection.

Azathioprine

Azathioprine is one of the cytotoxic drugs used to treat rheumatoid arthritis. It is generally introduced when other DMARDs, such as methotrexate and gold, have been ineffective.

Azathioprine acts to reduce cell proliferation, decrease the immune response, and reduce the amount of chemical inflammation. Azathioprine has been approved by the FDA for the treatment of rheumatoid arthritis.

The drug is taken by mouth on a daily basis and effects are generally noted after 2 to 3 months.

Azathioprine has proved to be a relatively safe drug, although the incidence of side effects is 20% to 30%. The majority of these are easily reversible once the drug is stopped. Often they can be eradicated by simply reducing the dose of the drug.

Side Effects: The most common side effect is a reduced blood count; as with other medications with this side effect, blood tests should be checked regularly. Reduced white cell count may be associated with an increased risk of infection. Systemic symptoms, such as nausea, fatigue, and fever, are relatively common. Liver toxicity occurs but is rare. Skin rashes are relatively common but are generally not considered serious. The risk of malignancy with prolonged azathioprine therapy has been evaluated: rheumatoid arthritis patients appear to have a slightly increased risk of lymphoma. The majority of studies, however, do not appear to indicate any significantly increased additional cancer risk with azathioprine.

Sulfasalazine

Sulfasalazine is an important drug in the treatment of inflammatory bowel disease but has also been used for rheumatoid arthritis. It is more extensively used in Europe than North America. Recently, there has been increased interest in the use of sulfasalazine in the treatment of ankylosing spondylitis and psoriatic arthritis.

The mechanism of action of sulfasalazine is not clear, but it appears to have an affect on folic acid metabolism, much like methotrexate. It may also reduce levels of auto-antibodies and inhibit the production of certain prostaglandins.

Sulfasalazine is a medication taken by mouth. It should not be taken by anyone with an allergy to sulpha.

Side Effects: Side effects include nausea and loss of appetite, fever and malaise, skin rash with photosensitivity, and mouth ulcers. Reduced blood cell count can occur and should be monitored regularly.

Biologic Response Modifying Drugs

Tumor Necrosis Factor Antibody (Infliximab - Remicade)

This recently developed treatment for rheumatoid arthritis and other inflammatory conditions is an antibody to tumor-necrosis-factor-alpha (TNF-alpha), an important chemical in the inflammatory process. TNF-alpha is produced in large quantities in rheumatoid arthritis and other conditions, such as psoriatic arthritis and inflammatory bowel disease. The antibody neutralizes the chemical and deactivates some of the cell receptors through which it acts.

In rheumatoid arthritis the combination treatment of methotrexate and infliximab is the only treatment approved by the FDA to improve physical function, inhibit progression of structural damage, and lessen signs and symptoms of the disease. It is indicated in patients with moderate to severe rheumatoid arthritis who have not responded or failed to continue to respond to methotrexate alone. The approval is based on a large double blind placebo controlled trial.

TNF-alpha antibody is usually infused intravenously over a 1- to 2-hour time period. Most patients show a significant improvement in symptoms within 48 hours. Unfortunately, approximately 10% of patients get an infusion reaction, which includes hives, shortness of breath, and reduced blood pressure. Supervision is therefore needed during infusions. Common side effects following infusion include coughs and colds, headaches, nausea, and skin rash. The treatment is contraindicated in patients with heart failure, history of tuberculosis, histoplasmosis, and certain neurologic conditions.

Etanercept (Enbrel)

Etanercept is classified along with infliximab as a biological response modifier. This injected medication binds to TNF-alpha and prevents its interaction with TNF receptors. Unlike the antibody infliximab, etanercept injection can be carried out by the patient and does not have to be intravenous. Supervision is not required, although there can be local reactions such as redness, swelling, and itching, as well as headaches and dizziness. It should not be given in the presence of co-existing infections. The annual cost is estimated at about $12,000 dollars. The injection is given as a twice-weekly subcutaneous injection.

Clinical studies are encouraging and show more rapid improvement of symptoms and reduced progression of joint damage than patients treated with oral methotrexate.

Leflunomide (Arava)

This oral medication works by inhibiting the proliferation of white cells at the site of inflammation and reducing the number of chemicals released to promote inflammation. In clinical trials, it is comparable in effectiveness to sulfasalazine and methotrexate. Unfortunately, the drug has a number of side effects, the most significant of which is liver damage and failure. Its use is contraindicated in patients with decreased liver function, although significant liver damage can occur even in normal individuals. The overall risk of liver damage is controversial but appears markedly increased when the drug is combined with methotrexate use.

Anakinra (Kineret)

Anakinra is an analogue of a human interleukin-1 receptor antagonist. This means it is a molecule that blocks the action of the cytokine inter leukin-1 (IL-1), one of the most important mediators of inflammation in arthritis. High levels of IL-1 are found in synovial fluid in rheumatoid arthritis, and it potentiates cartilage breakdown and bone resorption. Small amounts of the IL-1 blocker exist physiologically, but administration of the synthesized form markedly reduces inflammation and normalizes cartilage cell activity.

Anakinra is given by self injection under the skin, effects being noted at about 4 weeks. Its efficacy has been demonstrated in at least 3 clinical trials. About 70% of subjects will experience injection site reaction, but this is only serious enough to stop treatment in 7% to 10% of patients.

Antibiotic Therapy in Inflammatory Arthritis

While no specific transmissible infectious organisms have been identified as a pathogenic cause of rheumatoid arthritis, treatment of the disease with antibiotics has shown limited success (see minocycline). Rifamycin, an antibiotic inhibiting protein synthesis and used in the treatment of tuberculosis, has been found to be beneficial in inflammation of the knee in rheumatoid arthritis. Treatment with tetracycline has met with limited success. Other antibiotics include ceftriaxone and ampicillin. It is not yet clear whether these antibiotics target a causative organism or whether they target organisms that aggravate or increase progression of the disease or indeed whether they act through a different mechanism to alter the disease process. Research continues in this field.

Minocycline

Minocycline is an antibiotic in the tetracycline group. Although no transmissible pathogenic organism has been found to be associated with rheumatoid arthritis, minocycline has been found in early clinical trials to be an effective treatment for reducing inflammation and joint swelling.

The precise mechanism of action of minocycline is unclear. There is a suggestion that the organism mycoplasma may be a contributing factor in the development of inflammation in rheumatoid arthritis but studies are far from conclusive. Minocycline has also been shown to inhibit enzymes active in rheumatoid and other forms of arthritis that are responsible for joint destruction. Other proposed mechanisms of action include reduced prostaglandin production and reduced white cell activity and proliferation.

Early results of use of the drug minocylcine are interesting but not conclusive enough for it to be used as a standard medication. Benefits seem to occur mostly in patients with less severe forms of rheumatoid arthritis and most only show moderate improvement in symptoms.

Antibiotic Treatment in Septic Arthritis

Treatment of the acutely infected joint involves aggressive management, including splinting for pain relief, intravenous antibiotics, and surgical drainage. It has been suggested that in superficial joints, such as the knee, repeated removal of the infected fluid from the joint using a needle can be used as an alternative to surgery. However, this generally leaves pockets of infection and the results are not as reliable.

Antibiotic treatment is based initially on the most commonly suspected organisms, and is generally broad spectrum (aimed at a wide range of bacteria). Once test and culture results are known, more specific antibiotics are used. Antibiotic treatment in septic arthritis is often prolonged, lasting 6 or more weeks. During this time, use of the supplement acidophilus will help reduce the side effects of diarrhea, mouth ulceration, and yeast infections.

Surgical treatment involves thorough washing out and cleaning of the joint either through arthroscopy or open surgery. Arthroscopically amenable joints include the ankle, knee, hip, elbow, wrist, and shoulder. This treatment is generally successful in controlling the infection. Rarely is a second procedure required. In the presence of bone involvement or spread of the infection into the surrounding tissues, arthroscopy is not reliable and an open surgical procedure should be used. Open surgical procedures are also used in cases were the equipment or expertise is not available to carry out an arthroscopic procedure.

For gonococcal arthritis, treatment involves high dose intravenous or intramuscular antibiotics. The response is usually dramatic. Surgical treatment is not usually required, but removal of fluid from the joint may be required for diagnosis.

Injection Therapy

Injection therapy involves the introduction of a medication directly into an affected joint. If there is a substantial amount of fluid within the joint, this may be removed prior to injection of the medicine. There are two main medications, cortisone and hyaluronan.

Cortisone

Cortisone injections are generally used to alleviate acute pain and swelling in a joint that has not responded to treatment with oral medicine and such modalities as ice. Cortisone is an anti-inflammatory medication. It is a steroid, but is generally given as a formulation that results in no significant absorption into the circulation. Besides a temporary increase in blood sugar levels in susceptible individuals, cortisone injection into the joints is not associated with the systemic effects of cortisone taken by mouth or intramuscular injections. It acts locally to reduce the inflammatory response that is occurring in the lining of the joint. It is this inflammation that is responsible for much of the pain, swelling, stiffness, and dysfunction.

The procedure is straightforward. It should be carried out with sterile equipment following sterile cleaning of the skin. In certain joints, particularly where removal of fluid is going to be attempted (the knee, for example), a small injection of local anaesthetic into the skin and soft tissues can markedly reduce discomfort associated with the procedure. In general, if the physician is experienced, it is unusual for an injection of cortisone to be unduly painful. Mixing the cortisone (usually a long acting preparation) with some long acting anaesthetic can help reduce discomfort even further. In addition, the presence of the anaesthetic within the joint can often give immediate relief. This is a good indicator that the injection has been placed in the correct spot. Following the injection, vigorous activity is generally avoided for a few days. It is not uncommon to have some increased pain over the first 24 hours, perhaps as a reaction to the medication, but this usually subsides quite quickly. Regular icing following the injection will help minimize this.

One or two injections over a period of 4 to 6 weeks is reasonable, but frequent repeated injections increase joint damage and weaken the surrounding tissues.

Lumbar Epidural Injection

The injection of anti-inflammatory cortisone into the space surrounding the spinal cord and exiting nerve roots is referred to as an epidural injection. It aims to reduce the local inflammation that surrounds nerves following damage from arthritis or disc herniation. It is normally performed under x-ray guidance to ensure accurate placement of the needle.

There are no controlled clinical studies to indicate that epidural injection is effective. It does work in some cases, but the wide range of causes of low back pain make assessment of its specific indications difficult.

Facet Joint Blocks

Injection of cortisone into joints for the treatment of arthritis is a well-recognized and often effective form of treatment. Facet joint injection aims to place the cortisone into the inflamed arthritic facet joints of the posterior part of the spine. In theory, it seems like a good idea, but studies show the procedure to be no more effective than placebo in the treatment of low back pain. Again, this may be due to the multitude of causes of the condition, and the therapy could conceivably be beneficial in carefully selected cases.

Hyaluronan

Over the past few years, a number of products have been developed to replace hyaluronic acid (HA), a molecule in synovial fluid and articular cartilage. HA forms an essential part of the matrix 'glue' that binds articular joint cartilage together, attracting water and giving it structural properties to withstand the forces of joint impact and motion. It is also a critical component of the lubricating synovial joint fluid. In osteoarthritis, HA is found with decreased concentration and the molecules are smaller in size. This results in reduced lubrication and weaker cartilage. These injectable preparations of HA are classified as *devices* rather than drugs due to the proposed mechanical nature of their action.

The three main groups of HA are Low Molecular Weight (hyalgan and ARTZ); Medium Molecular Weight (orthovisc); and High Molecular Weight (synvisc). HA preparations need to be injected directly into the affected joint. They are most frequently used at the hip and the knee. In Canada, each injection costs about $100.00, though they are often covered by private insurance plans. Normally a series of three injections is used.

Laboratory trials of HA seem to indicate increased efficiency and mechanical properties with higher molecular weight. There is evidence that HA may inhibit the progression of osteoarthritis, induce cartilage development, and reduce fibrosis. In rheumatoid arthritis, it may be useful in reducing inflammation, as it appears to suppress the production of prostaglandin PGE-2.

Numerous clinical trials have now been carried out on the effectiveness of HA preparations. A Canadian multi-center trial in 1995 found HA to be a safe and effective treatment for osteoarthritis, either as a replacement or an adjunct to NSAID therapy. A randomized double blind placebo controlled clinical trial in the archives of internal medicine found that for resting pain relief HA was as affective as NSAIDs, and for pain associated with activity HA appeared to be superior. Hyaluronan treatment seems to be most effective in patients with earlier osteoarthritis. It has been considered inadvisable to treat patients with complete collapse of the joint or bone loss as their response is poor. HA injection also appears to be useful in rheumatoid arthritis, where at least some of its effect is mediated by a reduction in PGE-2.

Adverse affects from HA injection are reported in between 2% and 15% of patients. In most cases, this is local swelling and inflammation, although in some cases it can be quite severe. Infection secondary to injection is extremely rare but increases with the number of injections. Clearly, sterile technique must be used at all times.

Injectable hyaluronic acid therapy appears to be beneficial in some individuals with mild to moderate osteoarthritis and in rheumatoid arthritis. It may be considered as an alternative or adjunct to NSAID therapy and when other conservative modalities have failed. Studies thus far have shown benefit up to 6 months.

SURGICAL TREATMENTS FOR ARTHRITIS

Surgery for arthritis should be considered a last resort, used when other less invasive measures no longer control the symptoms of arthritis, such as pain, stiffness, and reduced function. Surgery for arthritis is not life saving but rather *lifestyle* saving. Arthritis surgery does not have to be performed: surgery is a choice made by the patient and the surgeon based on the severity of symptoms and the expectations of the patient. Invariably, this becomes an individual decision. Patients vary greatly in their expectations and requirements for lifestyle. One individual may request surgery to enable a return to the golf course, while another may not decide on the procedure until almost confined to the house due to pain and immobility.

The decision to undergo surgery should never be taken lightly. Even the simplest procedures carry with them some associated risks. However, with improvement in techniques of anaesthesia and advances in surgery, more often than not, the benefits of the procedure far outweigh the risks. Most patients are, not surprisingly, frightened of undergoing surgery. They have often heard unfortunate tales from friends about disastrous results and are often concerned that they may "never walk again." Unfortunately, rumors in the community are reported on much the same basis as newspapers and television. The vast majority of excellent results and happy patients never make it to the front page. Healthcare practitioners need to give patients accurate information on the options available to them, along with accurate data on their results. Only then can the patient make an informed decision about whether to go ahead with surgical treatment.

Arthroscopy (Arthroscopic Surgery)

Arthroscopy is a minimally invasive surgical technique used to evaluate and treat problems within certain joints. Since its introduction into North America in the early 1970s, the technique has revolutionized the management of many joint disorders. It is now the most commonly performed orthopedic procedure.

While the knee is still the most frequently 'scoped' joint, the shoulder is rapidly gaining ground. The elbow, ankle, hip, wrist, and temperomandibular joint of the jaw can also be accessed by arthroscopy for treatment of certain conditions.

The principal advantage of arthroscopy is that it results in minimal destruction of the structures surrounding a joint. It provides a far more desirable alternative to an arthrotomy, in which the whole joint is opened through an extensive incision. Arthroscopy is carried out through a series of small 'stab' incisions, often only 2-3 mm long. Scarring both outside and within the joint is minimized, allowing rapid recovery, rehabilitation, and return to function.

Arthroscopy is typically an outpatient procedure; that is, you remain in hospital for only a few hours. This is often referred to as day-surgery. Under most circumstances, you will not need to stay overnight. Arthroscopy does need to be performed in a hospital setting because it requires sterile conditions, anaesthetics, and often fairly complex equipment. This surgery may be performed under general anaesthetic, regional anaesthetic (in which an entire area of the body is anaesthetized), and occasionally under local anaesthesia. Local anaesthesia, involving simple freezing of the skin and within the joint, is often not practical, as the patient is not relaxed, tends to move around, and still feels pain from certain aspects of the joint and the procedure.

Once suitable anaesthesia is obtained, the outside of the joint is cleaned with antibacterial solution and covered with sterile sheets, leaving the joint exposed. The joint may be inflated with salt water or anaesthetic before the arthroscope is inserted through a small stab incision. The arthroscope is comprised of a rigid tube containing fiberoptic fibers to transmit light into the joint and a series of lenses to focus the image onto an eyepiece. In the early days of arthroscopy, the surgeon would look directly into the eyepiece, but with modern technology, a miniature camera can be fitted to the eyepiece to transmit the image to a monitor. Videotape, still pictures, or digital recordings can be incorporated into the circuit to allow a record of the pathology and surgery. The arthroscope can be moved around the joint and transferred to other portals to allow visualization of the entire joint. It is actually surprising that a far better view is obtained with the arthroscope in most instances than by opening up the joint with a large incision.

Second and third incisions or portals are made to allow drainage and access by other arthroscopic instruments. These instruments include small scissors, graspers, biters, and motorized shavers. They are used to treat the damage structures within the joint.

At the completion of the procedure, the joint is washed with salt water, the instruments removed and the incisions closed, usually with just one stitch. Bandages are applied and the patient is transferred to the recovery room and back to the day surgery unit. Once they are feeling comfortable, they are generally discharged home. Recovery from arthroscopic surgery is generally rapid but does vary considerably between patients, depending on the joint involved and the surgery performed.

Typical post-operative instructions for a patient undergoing knee arthroscopy are given below:

Post Operative Instructions

The following is a brief description of what was found in your knee and what surgery was carried out. I will discuss this more fully with you at your first clinic visit in 2 weeks:

1. _____

2. _____

INSTRUCTIONS

Dressing (Bandages)

Try not to remove the dressing for 48 hours unless your foot and ankle become swollen or begin to tingle. After this time, the bandage can be removed and the padding discarded. Try to leave the band-aids intact or apply new ones. Reapply the bandage and continue to wear it until the swelling subsides and the knee feels comfortable. Apply ice regularly to the knee (ice pack wrapped in towel for 15 - 20 minutes), starting on the evening of surgery. Remove the tensor bandage and reapply it whenever it feels too tight, your foot and ankle swell, or you feel tingling in the foot.

Showering

You may shower 48 hours after surgery. Replace the band-aids with fresh ones afterwards. Do not soak in a bath or whirlpool or go swimming until the stitches have been removed. You will have instructions to have the stitches removed by your Family Doctor in 10 to 14 days or when you return to the clinic.

Activity

Start immediately with straight leg lifts and try to so at least 200 per day. Bend the knee as much as possible without pain. Walk, climb stairs, cycle, and try to resume normal activity as soon as possible. Return to school/office work in 2 to 3 days, heavy manual work in 3 to 4 weeks, and sports in 2 to 3 weeks.

Analgesics

You will be given a prescription for painkillers. Use them as needed. For less pain, use plain tylenol. Use ice as described above in addition to painkillers. Eat plenty of bran/fiber and drink prune juice, as the pain pills may cause constipation.

Follow-up

Please call my office and book an appointment with my secretary for two weeks following the surgery.

Arthroscopy has revolutionized treatment of the arthritic joint, particularly the knee. It allows assessment and surgical treatment of the joint with rapid recovery and minimal side effects. It has filled an important gap between non-surgical treatments, such as medications and injections, and the more extensive surgical procedures, such as total joint replacement, which involve more extensive hospitalization, prolonged recovery, and greater potential complications.

Suitability of Treatment

Unfortunately, arthroscopy does not provide the surgical solution to arthritis in all individuals. The following factors may influence your suitability for this treatment:

Joint Involved

With respect to the joint involved in the arthritis, there are two factors. One is accessibility by the arthroscope and the second is the ability to identify and treat arthritic damage that is likely to result in an improvement in symptoms. The knee is the best example of a joint that is easily accessed by the arthroscope and often contains significant treatable pathology; however, the hip is very inaccessible and treatable pathology is difficult to assess. There are few centers that have reported success in the treatment of this joint, and, in general, it is not routinely performed. The shoulder is very accessible via arthroscopy, but there is usually less treatable pathology than in the knee. Arthritis in the shoulder does not usually cause problems until it is quite severe, and, at this point, arthroscopic treatment is usually not helpful. Synovectomy (see below) may be helpful in the patient with inflammatory arthritis, but this is technically a difficult procedure in the shoulder. The elbow and ankle are equally accessible, but treatment is usually confined to the removal of loose fragments of bone, bone spurs, and synovium. Results are variable. Arthritis of the spine is not accessible via the arthroscope.

Severity of Arthritis

In general, the more severe the arthritis, the more unpredictable the outcome of arthroscopic surgery. There are certain patients we see for whom we do not feel arthroscopy is worth attempting due to the severity of the degenerative change in the joint. Normally, at the knee, this would involve extensive collapse of the bone with deformity and bone-on-bone arthritis.

Type of Arthritis

Arthroscopic treatment of inflammatory arthritis is generally more successful if it is performed early on and combined with synovectomy. The more advanced the changes and damage within the joint, the less effective arthroscopy is. With osteoarthritis, the procedure can be performed at any time, but the more severe the changes, the less predictable the outcome.

Previous Procedures

Repeat arthroscopy generally follows a law of diminishing return. Certainly, if an individual has had relief of pain, swelling, and mechanical symptoms for a year or two, then repeating the procedure can be beneficial. If, however, the results have only lasted a few weeks, then a repeat procedure is almost certain to fail. There are, of course, exceptions to this rule, such as when new pathology has developed following a repeat injury, for example, but this is uncommon.

Types of Arthoscopic Surgery

Arthroscopic Debridement

This procedure refers to the evaluation of a joint with arthroscopy and the treatment of damaged areas within the joint. It can be considered a 'spring clean up' or 'lube, oil and filter'. During the procedure, synovial joint fluid and debris is washed from the joint. Areas of cartilage damage can be smoothed down. Specific areas of inflammation in the lining can be removed. Loose fragments of bone or cartilage can be removed and bony spurs that are rubbing on tissues or causing restrictions to movement can be trimmed or removed. In the knee, the meniscal cartilages can be trimmed as they show wear and damage with age. Tidying up of a degenerative meniscal cartilage in the absence of any other areas of significant arthritis it is often extremely successful.

Arthroscopic debridement does not cure arthritis. It aims to improve the symptoms that are caused by the arthritis, such as pain, swelling, catching or locking, and a feeling of weakness. In general, the symptoms tend to come back eventually, but the time frame can be quite variable. Good results are reported in 50% to 80% of patients at 2 to 4 years. On average, about 70% of patients can expect relief of pain at 2 years following the procedure. These results, however, vary considerably with patient age and the severity of the arthritis. Discussion with your surgeon will determine whether you are a candidate for arthroscopic debridement, and if so, the likelihood of it being successful.

Arthroscopic Synovectomy

The synovium or lining of the joint is an important part of the disease process in inflammatory arthritis, such as rheumatoid arthritis. Changes in the synovium often occur before there is any damage to the joint, joint surface, or surrounding structures. The synovium produces vast amounts of damaging chemicals and enzymes, and is itself invasive, causing erosions and damage to the bone around the joint. For this reason, the surgical technique of synovectomy was developed. Removal of this aggressive tissue results in reduced pain and swelling, reduced stiffness, and decreased joint destruction.

Synovectomy was originally performed in most joints through an open procedure, and this is still required in certain cases and certain joints. In the elbow, for example, where removal of the synovium is often associated with removal of the head of the radius, the procedure is probably more easily accomplished through an open incision. With regards to the knee, arthroscopic synovectomy provides an excellent alternative to the open operation. The technique is performed in much the same way as a regular arthroscopy (see above), but a larger number of portals are made in order to access the different areas of the joint. There is usually a significant amount of bleeding, and a surgical drain is often left in the joint for a few hours to avoid build-up of a large blood clot. These procedures are generally performed with an overnight stay in hospital. The risk of infection is somewhat higher than from a regular arthroscopy, and as a result antibiotics are usually given.

Arthroscopic synovectomy is used predominantly in inflammatory arthritis where excess synovial proliferation plays a more active role in the disease process. However, in certain cases it can also be beneficial in osteoarthritis. The procedure is performed when medication therapy has failed, and works best before there is evidence of bone and cartilage damage on x-rays. Results of arthroscopic synovectomy in the knee are encouraging with 75% to 80% of patients reporting reduction in pain and swelling at 2 to 4 years.

Complications of Knee Arthroscopy

Complications of arthroscopy are uncommon. The majority of them are minor, easily treatable, and unlikely to result in any permanent problems.

Haemarthrosis (1%)

Bleeding into the joint is more common after arthroscopic debridement for arthritis, and, in particular, following synovectomy. Drainage may be required if severe (0.2%).

Blood Clot (Thrombosis) (0.1%)

Clots in the deep veins of the leg are very uncommon due to the brief immobility and minimally invasive surgery. Calf pain and swelling should be checked and an ultrasound test carried out if there is any suspicion. In rare cases where a blood clot occurs, anti-coagulation treatment is required for 3 to 6 months.

Pulmonary Embolus (0.025%)

This is where a clot from the leg breaks off and goes to the lungs. It is extremely rare. Chest pain or shortness of breath are warning signs and should be immediately evaluated by your doctor. Treatment is with blood-thinners.

Infection (0.1%)

About 1 in 1000 individuals get an infection after arthroscopy. This may be just a small skin infection around one of the portal incisions, but occasionally it involves the inside of the joint. Pain, heat, redness, and swelling associated with malaise and fever are warning signs. Treatment may involve withdrawal of fluid for testing and repeat arthroscopy to wash out the infection. Antibiotic treatment for 4 to 6 weeks is usually required. Overall, recovery is usually excellent, with no long-term problems once the inflammation and stiffness has resolved.

Nerve Injury

Major nerve injury is exceedingly rare. Tiny skin nerves around the knee can be damaged by the incisions leading to very small areas of numbness. These are rarely bothersome.

Arthrotomy (Open Debridement)

As opposed to arthroscopic examination, an arthrotomy involves an incision made over a joint to allow direct access. Having done this, the joint can be accessed and cleaned much as with the arthroscopic procedure. The advantages of this procedure are that a wider range of joints can be accessed and that more aggressive removal of bone can be carried out. Open synovectomy may also be carried out at the same procedure. The procedure is often carried out at the first metatarsophalangeal joint at the base of the great toe. Individuals developing arthritis at this site develop what is called hallux rigidus or a stiff toe. There is often pain from bone spurs around the joint, particularly on pushing off from the ground. Removal of these bone spurs and cleaning up of the joint is often a very successful procedure. Open debridement of the ankle and elbow often allow removal of large bone spurs that are causing pain, catch in certain positions, or restrict movement.

Arthrodesis (Fusion of a Joint)

As a joint becomes more and more severely arthritic, its movement becomes progressively more restricted. In some cases, the restriction of movement may become so severe that the joint remains stuck in one position. This joint is considered fused or arthrodesed. Once a joint has reached this state, it often becomes less painful. Much of the pain from arthritis appears to come from the movement of two damaged surfaces across each other, and this no longer happens in the fused joint.

Surgical arthrodesis or fusion is a procedure by which the joint is fused earlier in order to eliminate pain. This technique was used quite extensively in the early days of orthopedic surgery but has become less and less popular with the development of newer techniques, in particular, joint replacement. However, it still has a certain role in certain joints and situations.

Surgical arthrodesis is most commonly employed in the spine. By creating a bony bridge across segments of the spine, movement can be eliminated, thereby relieving pain from the disc and the small facet joints. Fusion is very rarely used in such joints as the hip or knee, except as a salvage procedure in cases where other techniques, including joint replacement, have failed. It may be required following severe infection where use of a joint replacement would be contraindicated. The most commonly fused joint is probably the ankle. Pain and stiffness seem to go hand in hand, such that by the time a patient requires such extensive surgery to deal with the pain, much of the movement is already lost. The procedure has a high success rate and seems to be well tolerated by patients. Modification of shoe wear is generally required after the surgery. The reason why ankle fusion remains popular is the lack of a proven joint replacement at this site. Early attempts to replace the joint were fraught with early failure. While newer designs look promising, their survival needs to be established before they are used routinely. Fusion is also used extensively in the hands and feet where loss of movement is more easily accommodated.

Fusion of a joint generally requires an open surgical procedure, although some reports indicate the procedure being performed through the arthroscope. Often bone graft is required, and the joint usually needs to be fixed with screws or plates supported with an external cast for a number of weeks.

Osteotomy (Realignment of the Joint)

The technique of surgical osteotomy refers to the realignment of a bone above or below a joint in order to change the forces across the joint. Generally, the procedure is carried out to unload a damaged area of the joint. For example, in the knee, if the inner part is damaged resulting in a bowleg deformity, then the shinbone or tibia can be surgically realigned such that the force in the knee passes through the outer compartment. This procedure is called a high-tibial-osteotomy.

Osteotomy procedures are used almost exclusively at the hip and the knee, but their use has diminished considerably over the past 20 years with the increasing success and indication for joint replacement. Osteotomy procedures still have an important role, particularly in the younger individual who may, for example, still be employed in heavy work, which would induce too much wear on a joint replacement. Recovery from an osteotomy may take longer than a joint replacement as the realigned bone needs to heal and the limb needs to readjust to its new alignment. Excellent results can be expected in appropriately selected patients, and, generally, these procedures continue to give good results for 8 to 10 years. At this time, the patient may well be ready for a total joint replacement. Joint replacement arthroplasty following osteotomy at the hip and the knee is technically more demanding, but the overall outcome does not appear to be significantly affected.

Joint Replacement Arthroplasty

The introduction of the total hip replacement arthroplasty procedure by Sir John Charnley in England in the mid 1960s initiated a revolution in orthopedic surgery that has gained momentum over the past 40 years. It is estimated that over 200,000 hip arthroplasties are performed annually in the United States; figures from 1988 showed that one million Americans had already undergone the procedure. Over 42,000 hip and knee replacements were performed in Canada in 1999-2000, an increase of 32% from 1994-1995. Nearly 90% of total joint replacements were in people over 55 years of age, with 60% being women. With an aging, active population these figures are only going to increase.

Our patient's often ask if they need a joint replacement. We tell them that only *they* can answer that question. Joint replacement surgery is not like surgery for a fracture or for cancer. In these cases, the surgery needs to be done to avoid potentially disastrous outcomes. With surgery for arthritis, the orthopedic surgeon is able to offer the procedure as a method of treatment and inform the patient of the potential benefits and associated risks, but the ultimate decision to go ahead lies with the patient. Joint replacement surgery, as in other forms of surgery for arthritis, is lifestyle saving rather than life saving.

Joint replacement surgery is a last resort, the final stage of treatment of arthritis, when all other forms of treatment have failed. When we see patients who are candidates for total joint replacement, we ensure that they have tried all other forms of treatment. We evaluate their level of dis-ability, such as the distance they can walk without pain, and their ability to carry out simple functions, such as cutting their toenails or bending and reaching in the garden. We examine their x-rays and any other tests that are available. We thoroughly explain the procedure, the hospital stay, the rehabilitation, and the average recovery milestones they can expect in the post-operative period. We discuss the possible complications of the procedure and how long the implant is likely to last. Having done all this, we usually leave them with a pamphlet, reiterating our discussion, and advise them to go home, think about the surgery, and discuss it with their family before calling back to confirm. They often return with relatives and friends to ask further questions before deciding on booking a date for the procedure.

Total joint replacement arthroplasty is one of the most successful oper-ations available today. It has been repeatedly proven to provide improve-ment not only in pain and mobility, but in overall quality and enjoyment of life. Consistently, 98% to 99% of patients get a good or excellent result, and serious complications are rare. Given this success rate, it saddens us to see otherwise healthy individuals disabled from arthritis and accepting a poor quality of life because of unwarranted fear of surgical intervention, generally due to misinformation by friends or health practitioners. Make sure you get all the facts from someone knowledgeable before making your decision.

Types of Total Joint Replacement

Total joint technology is a rapidly evolving field with innovative materials and designs being launched at a frantic rate. Caution should be exercised, however, as new is not necessarily better. Implants that appeared initially to have solved many problems have ended up being discarded because of unforeseen complications. Standard joint replacements available now have an excellent track record and generally predictable outcome, and this should not be sacrificed for the possibility for a yet unproven 'state-of-the-art' device.

Total Hip Replacement

The hip joint is the first joint to be successfully replaced using modern arthroplasty techniques, but since the pioneering work of Sir John Charnley in England with his low friction hip arthroplasty, there have been many developments in design and biomaterials. The most popular design for a total joint replacement is illustrated here. There are two components: the socket part, which is comprised of an outer metal shell with an inner lining of high-density low friction polyethylene; and the femoral component, which is comprised of a stem to be fixed securely inside the hollow canal of the upper thigh bone, topped with a polished metallic ball that fits into the plastic socket.

The orthopedic community continues to discuss, develop, and analyze different implants, but the two most common designs are the hybrid total hip replacement and the uncemented total hip replacement.

In the hybrid total hip replacement design, the acetabulum or cup side is metal with an outer porous surface that is wedged tightly into the prepared socket in the pelvis. The porous design allows for ingrowth of bone that holds the socket in place on a long-term basis. Within this outer metal shell, there is a plastic liner comprised of high-density polyethylene, which provides excellent wear and low friction characteristics. The femoral side of a hybrid total hip replacement is a metallic stem fixed into the thighbone with pressurized cement. This is the implant generally used in patients over 65 years of age and of standard build. It allows immediate full weight bearing following surgery and provides excellent pain relief. The device has shown great longevity.

In the uncemented total hip replacement design, the cup is the same as with the hybrid, but the femoral side is covered in porous material to allow ingrowth of bone to fix the implant. Initial stability is obtained by ensuring an extremely tight fit. This implant has the disadvantage that protected weight bearing is usually required for 4 to 6 weeks. This is needed to improve the ingrowth of bone and fixation of the stem. This type of implant is used extensively in younger individuals (below age 60), but its indications over recent years have been expanded to include older patients with good bone quality who are more active and of heavier build. Generally, this type of implant requires excellent bone quality for solid initial fixation and subsequent ingrowth. Development of thigh pain can occur in certain individuals and can be quite bothersome.

New developments in total hip arthroplasty include materials to reduce friction and wear. High density plastic for the socket appears to last longer

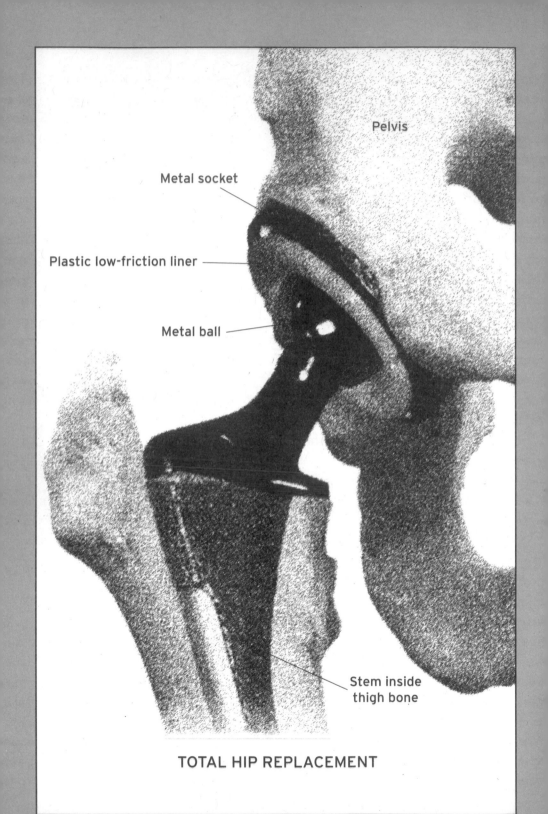

Pelvis

Metal socket

Plastic low-friction liner

Metal ball

Stem inside
thigh bone

TOTAL HIP REPLACEMENT

than previously tested materials. The development of ceramic heads resulted in decreased friction but greater fragility and a tendency for the hip to fracture. New developments in ceramic technology have allowed the heads to be made of smaller particles with somewhat reduced fracture risk. This problem, however, continues to be an issue with ceramic material. Metal bearings with no plastic liner do produce wear, but it has been suggested that the particles cause less inflammation than the plastic particles. These investigations are ongoing.

One of the newest developments is the minimally invasive surface replacement hip arthroplasty. Interestingly, this revisits a very old design of hip replacement abandoned with the advent of the total joint design. Structural redesign and new materials appear to have made this implant viable once again, but it is still largely experimental, being performed only in select locations and in selective cases.

Total Knee Replacement

Total knee replacement is the most common joint replacement performed. Unlike the hip joint, total joint replacement at the knee does not replace the entire joint, aiming to replace the surface of the joint only. The majority of the bone and its attached ligaments are kept intact. These are essential for proper functioning of the joint after surgery. The most popular total knee replacements incorporate a metal component over the end of the thigh bone that may be fixed by cement or by bony ingrowth and a metal tray that sits at the top of the shin bone with pegs or a stem through which it is fixed into the bone again, either with cement or bony ingrowth. Between the two sits a plastic spacer to provide friction-free motion. The under surface of the kneecap is also involved in the arthritis process and may or may not be resurfaced.

One of the most important recent developments in knee replacement arthroplasty is the redesign of the partial knee replacement. In select cases, only the inner or outer portion of the joint is significantly damaged and causing pain. One side of the joint can be replaced alone. This technique has been around for many years, but recently newer designs have allowed the procedure to be performed through a small incision. These are the so-called minimally invasive techniques. The advantage for the patient includes much reduced pain and a far more rapid recovery. While these

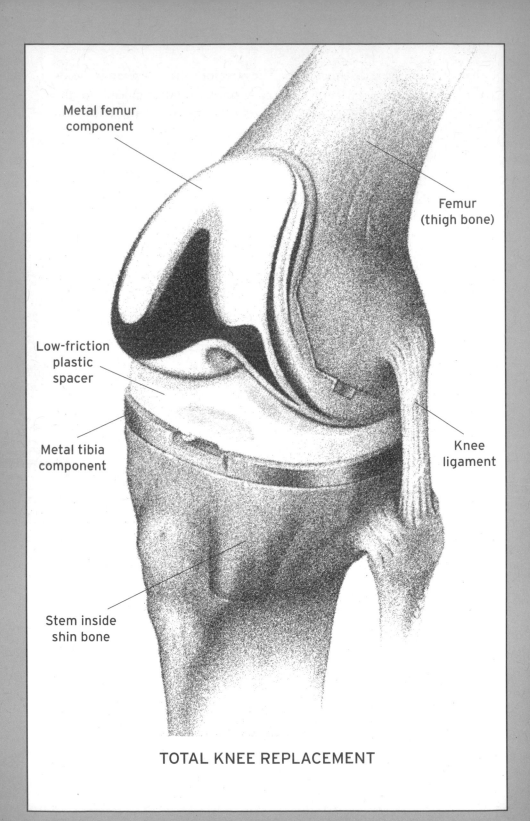

Metal femur
component

Femur
(thigh bone)

Low-friction
plastic
spacer

Metal tibia
component

Knee
ligament

Stem inside
shin bone

TOTAL KNEE REPLACEMENT

implants may seem like an excellent option, they are not designed for every-one. They will only work in selected patients with well-localized arthritis.

Total Shoulder Replacement

Osteoarthritis in the shoulder is uncommon and generally affects an older population than the hip or the knee. In many cases, it exists without sig-nificant symptoms. The shoulder is frequently involved in rheumatoid arthritis, with up to 60% of individuals with severe disease being affected at this joint. Although the shoulder is rarely the initial joint involved in rheumatoid arthritis, it tends to affect a younger population, typically women between 35 and 55 years of age.

Total shoulder replacement arthroplasty is performed much less com-monly than hip or knee replacement, simply because fewer patients afflicted by arthritis at this site have symptoms severe enough to warrant such intervention. However, when the procedure is carried out, the results are generally excellent. Over 90% of patients can expect to attain good or excellent pain relief. Restoration of range of motion is a little more variable and a number of factors come into play, including the severity of motion loss before the surgery, inflammation of the joint, and damage to the surrounding muscle.

Total shoulder replacement surgery follows a similar design to the hip with replacement of the ball and socket. The ball is usually replaced by a metallic head secured with a stem inside the bone at the upper end of the humerus. It is fixed with cement or with material to allow ingrowth of bone. The socket is usually all plastic and fixed with cement.

Early movement following total shoulder replacement is extremely important to minimize stiffness and maximize function. The shoulder is not a weight bearing joint, and complications related to wear are less fre-quent than at the hip or knee. The shoulder, however, is a complex joint and other complications can occur. The risk of a significant complication is estimated at 10% to 15%. One study reported excellent results (over 80% of normal motion) in 60% in cases and satisfactory results (at least half of normal range of motion) in 88% percent. Revision rates are low, averaging less than 5%.

Total Elbow Replacement

Osteoarthritis is most unusual at the elbow and rarely is severe enough to lead to a total elbow arthroplasty. It is most commonly seen in men with a history of heavy use of the arm. Post-traumatic arthritis can occur as a long-term result of fracture. The commonest diagnosis for which total elbow arthroplasty is carried out is rheumatoid arthritis. Although the joint is not one of the most commonly involved in rheumatoid arthritis, when it is, the pain, swelling, and dysfunction can be severely disabling. The elbow is a most essential joint because without it, use of the hand is severely limited.

The most commonly used elbow replacements today involve the so-called 'sloppy hinge'. These implants allow sufficient laxity of movement to prevent excessive strain on the implants and subsequent loosening.

The results from total elbow arthroplasty are excellent. Pain relief in over 90% of patients is to be expected, comparable to the results for total hip and knee replacements. Restoration of range of motion is predictable, even in patients with severe stiffness before surgery. Improvements in strength and function are tremendous. The most commonest causes of failure are loosening, dislocation, and infection.

Total Ankle Replacement

Early results with total ankle replacements were extremely discouraging, leading to near abandonment of the procedure and a return to the tried and tested operation of ankle fusion. Recent developments in materials and biomechanics have shown promise with respect to new designs for replacement of the ankle joint in osteoarthritis, post-traumatic arthritis, and rheumatoid arthritis.

In the original designs, all components were fixed, which resulted in too much loosening and subsequent failure. The new designs incorporate a mobile plastic bearing that is not fixed and thus greatly reduces friction. Early results indicate an 85% success rate. The procedure is still in development, and further studies need to be done before it becomes generally available.

The Procedure

Once you and your surgeon have decided upon a date for the joint replacement surgery, there will likely be a further explanation and discussion of the type of replacement to be used and a reiteration of potential complications before going ahead with signing of a consent form. If you have any medical problems, then your surgeon may arrange for you to be reviewed by an internist to evaluate your heart and lungs to ensure that there are no increased risk factors that need to be addressed before your surgery. This doctor will generally follow you during your stay in hospital, along with your orthopedic surgeon, in the event that there are any medical problems. An anaesthesiologist, who will be able to discuss your options for anaesthesia and pain relief for the procedure, may also evaluate you. You will likely need a visit to the hospital for some blood tests and an ECG (heart tracing), and for an educational session with a nurse or physiotherapist.

The Day of Surgery

On the day of surgery, you are generally required to be in the hospital about 2 hours before your procedure. You must have nothing to eat or drink that day. You will be admitted to hospital and transferred to a preparation ward. Here, you will be asked to change into a gown and an intravenous will be started through which the antibiotics that are to be used to cover your procedure will be given. Once you get to the operating room, you will meet the surgeon and the anaesthetist. The joint to be operated on will be marked clearly. As a general rule, orthopedic surgeons like to operate through their initials as one of the many checks to ensure that the correct limb is operated upon.

Once inside the operating room, you will either have a general anaesthetic or a regional anaesthetic, such as a spinal. Spinal anaesthetics can generally be used for hip and knee surgery. Some centers prefer regional blocks for shoulder surgery and elbow surgery as well, but this is a little less common. The joint to be operated upon will then be cleaned and sterilized before being covered with protective sheets. The surgeon will then perform the surgery with one or two other doctors providing assistance. There will a scrub nurse assisting with the procedure and one or two other nurses in the room to help ensure all equipment is available.

At the completion of the procedure, you will be sent to the recovery room. Here you will awake from a general anaesthetic or stabilized with your spinal anaesthetic before returning to your ward. Your surgeon will come and check on you before going to meet with any members of your family who might be waiting, to let them know that things went well. Your doctor will normally visit you a little later in the day upon on the ward and will generally visit once per day to ensure that things are going smoothly. If there are any problems at other times, your doctor will be contacted by the nursing staff looking after you by telephone.

Hospital Stay

There is tremendous variation in the duration of hospital stays. In Canada, you will usually be in hospital for 5 to 7 days before being transferred to a rehabilitation hospital. In other centers, you might be transferred a little earlier, and in some instances, transferred home for physiotherapy there.

During the first 24 to 48 hours, you will generally have your highest level of discomfort. If you have had spinal anaesthetic, this will likely last about 8 to 12 hours. If you have a spinal anaesthetic with a catheter left in place (epidural catheter), you will generally remain pain-free until this has been removed. It can be kept in for a number of days. In some cases, you may be given injections of painkillers by nursing staff or you may be provided with a pump through which you can administer your own medication. These pumps are carefully controlled so it is not possible for you to overdose (patient controlled anaesthesia or PCA).

Generally, the physiotherapist will encourage you get up and take a few steps even on the first day. Your surgeon will have left instructions as to how much weight you are allowed to put through the operated leg if it is a hip or knee replacement. In about 48 hours, you will generally have the dressings changed and any drains removed. Movement of the joint begins almost immediately in most cases. A machine may be used, particularly on the knee (CPM or continuous passive motion machine), to assist you in restoring movement. It is important to get the joint moving early before it begins to stiffen.

After a few days, you will generally be able to move independently, and at this stage, you are ready to be transferred to rehabilitation. Rehabilitation hospitals should not be thought of as a standard acute care hospital. You are encouraged to return to as normal a life as possible and will participate in numerous exercises along with many others who have had the same or similar procedure. It is designed to prepare you to go back home. During your stay at rehabilitation, there will generally be a doctor looking after you, and this may be an orthopedic surgeon. If it is not your surgeon, then the doctor at the rehabilitation hospital will generally stay in touch with the surgeon and will transfer you back to your surgeon's care if there are any untoward problems.

By the time you are discharged from rehabilitation, you will generally have been assessed for outpatient physiotherapy and been seen by an occupational therapist who will have instituted some devices and aides to assist with your day-to-day living at home.

We generally see our total joint replacement arthroplasties within 4-6 weeks following surgery, providing there are no problems or complications that cause them to come back sooner.

Recovery Expectations

Most patients, between 98% and 99%, are happy with their joint replacement. They can expect to be pain-free apart from perhaps the occasional twinge or ache when the weather changes. They can expect to have a good range of motion, allowing them to participate in most day-to-day activities. There is often better range of motion than before surgery and improved level of function. With respect to hip and knee replacements, patients should expect unrestricted walking tolerance, ability to perform household chores and gardening, and the ability to participate in certain sports. It is extremely important for you to discuss your expectations with your surgeon before the procedure. If your surgeon is expecting you to have a pain-free knee with good movement allowing you to tend the garden and play a round of golf, and you are expecting to compete in the next Boston Marathon, then clearly this discrepancy needs to be cleared up prior to surgery.

All patients are different, and the recovery and outcome of joint replacement surgery is very dependent on a number of factors, including pre-existing level of health and fitness. A brand new total knee is not going to allow someone with heart failure to do more exercise than they could before the surgery. It will, however, allow them to do the same amount without pain.

Current hip and knee replacements should last 10 to 15 years as a conservative estimate. This figure, however, depends greatly on the activity of the patient, and this is often related to age. Patients in their seventies who enjoy simple walking might reasonably expect to have their replacement last 15 to 20 years. A 55-year-old who decides to return to playing squash and takes up running may not make it to 10 years. There are number of other factors with respect to the type of implant used and the methods used to fix it that may influence survival.

Complications of Total Joint Replacement

Surgical Complications

Blood Loss

Performing a total joint replacement in the larger joints such as hips, knees, or shoulders is quite an extensive procedure and invariably results in some loss of blood. Even when surgery in the knee is performed with a tourniquet to prevent blood loss during the procedure, there will be blood loss afterwards, which is usually drained from the joint through a small drain. Precautions will be taken to ensure that blood loss is kept to a minimum, but even so, your blood level (haemoglobin) will be checked during the post-operative period to make sure that is has not dropped dangerously low. You will often be started on an iron supplement to allow your body to start manufacturing new blood cells.

In general, if your blood level drops low enough to pose a significant risk to your health, you will be considered for a blood transfusion. Your surgeon will usually discuss with you the possibility of blood loss before the surgery and you should make it clear if you do not want to receive one under any circumstances. Currently, the risks of receiving a blood transfusion are exceedingly small and likely less than the risks to your general health from not having one.

In some institutions it is possible to recycle the blood that is lost during and after the procedure and give it back to you. You should ask your doctor if this is available to you.

Infection

The risk of infection following your surgery is less than 1%. You will be given antibiotics to cover the operation and for a short time afterwards. Nevertheless, infections do occasionally occur. This may be a simple infection affecting the skin and incision and will be treated just with antibiotics.

More serious deep infections would generally require a further surgery with cleaning out of the joint. With these early infections it is not usually necessary to remove the joint replacement.

Venous Thrombosis

Following hip or knee replacement, the incidence of blood clots in the legs (deep venous thrombosis or DVT) would be very high were it not for treatment with blood-thinners. Without preventive treatment as many as 80% of hip and knee joint replacement patients would develop a venous thrombosis, and of these, between 10% and 20% would develop a pulmonary embolism in which a small fragment of the clot in the leg breaks off and goes to the lungs.

Prevention is achieved through early mobilization of the patient and an active exercise regime. Compression stockings may be applied to the legs to improve blood circulation. Most importantly, blood-thinning medications are used around the time of surgery and for a short period afterwards to reduce the risk. With these measures, the risk of a significant thrombosis that requires further treatment is less than 5% and the risk of a pulmonary embolus less than 1%.

Nerve and Artery Damage

The risk of damage to a major nerve or artery is exceedingly low. Some tiny skin nerves are unavoidable when making the surgical incision, and this may result in a small area of numbness around the scar. This is generally most noticeable at the knee. This area will generally get smaller over time, and it is very unusual for it to remain bothersome.

General Complications

General complications that occur around the time of any surgery include infections of the chest or bladder, which require antibiotic treatment. More elderly patients may develop a short period of confusion, which results from a combination of an altered environment and the medications that are required for anaesthesia and pain relief. Generally, this is brief and resolves quickly. At particular risk are individuals who drink alcohol on a daily basis. Serious health risks associated with surgery include heart attack and stroke but these occur extremely rarely. If you are at a significantly higher risk, this will be evaluated and discussed with you before surgery.

Early Post-Operative Complications

These complications generally occur in the first few weeks following the surgery. They may occur at the rehabilitation hospital or on discharge home from attending regular physiotherapy.

Venous Thrombosis

This can occur up to 3 months following your surgery but the highest risk is generally within the first 10 days.

Infection

Acute infection can occur within the first few weeks following surgery. A severe infection within the joint will require re-operation with cleaning of the joint. Even at this early stage, if the replacement remains securely fixed, it can often be left in place while the infection is treated with clean-out surgery and antibiotics.

Stiffness

The post-operative period is an extremely important time for restoring movement. Immediately following the surgery your body will want to produce scar tissue and restrict movement in the joint. This can occur at all joints but is particularly bothersome in the shoulder, elbow, and knee. Trying your best with the exercise program and using the CPM machine will certainly help.

We often tell our patients that every few degrees gained in the first week after surgery is worth at least 20 degrees at 6 weeks. Occasionally, despite their best efforts, patients find their joints are just too stiff and painful to move. They may then be a candidate for a *manipulation*. If we see a patient for the first post-operative visit for their total knee replacement at 4 weeks and they still have not achieved 90 degrees bend and have plateaued with their therapy, then we will recommend a manipulation. This is not a surgical procedure but involves a few moments of anaesthesia. Once asleep, we generally find the patient's knee bends up quite easily. A few bands of scar tissue are felt to pop and the knee is immediately placed on the CPM machine. Most patients find this extremely beneficial and go on to achieve an excellent range of motion.

Dislocation

This is generally only a problem in the hip joint. Great care is taken to ensure that muscles are appropriately tensioned and that it is very difficult for the hip to slip out of joint. If you have had a hip replacement, you will be advised on certain maneuvers that should be avoided, for example, crossing your legs or bending your hip more than 90 degrees. Although certain precautions are recommended on a long-term basis, they must be strictly adhered to during the first 6 weeks after the surgery.

Late Complications

Late complications can occur in the months and years following your joint replacement. With recent advances in design, materials, and techniques, many late complications, such as implant failure and loosening, have been minimized. The risk remains, estimated at about 1% per year.

Infection

Infection can occur at any time. It is important that you tell any other treating doctors or dentists about your joint implant. Generally, for procedures that are likely to lead to a release of bacteria into the blood stream (dental work, bowel or bladder surgery), you will require antibiotics. The usual recommendation is clindamycin 300 mg by mouth 1 hour before the procedure and 150 mg, 6 hours later.

Late infection often doesn't present with sudden pain and swelling. It can present as a gradual loosening of the implant with erosion of bone. This will result in increased pain in the joint. Following investigation, if you do have an infection, you will need further surgery. Although, in some cases, the infected implant can be removed and new one placed at the same operation, as a rule there is a 6-week interval during which treatment with antibiotics is continued before the new joint replacement inserted.

Loosening without Infection

Total joint replacements are fixed securely at the time of insertion, with cement or with a tight fit allowing in-growth of your own bone to secure the prosthesis. Loosening can occur for a number of reasons besides infection. Wear particles from the joint may cause inflammation that results in loosening. Deterioration and cracking in the cement may cause it to crumble and loosen the implant. A loose implant that is causing pain or erosion of the bone will generally need to be changed or revised. The old implant is removed and a new implant is inserted. On occasion, this can be quite straightforward, but in some circumstances a more complex reconstruction may be required. If a loose implant is identified, it is generally better to have it revised because progressive loosening carries with it a risk of bone fracture and bone loss that would make revision surgery more complicated. Considerable orthopedic research is now aimed at minimizing these complications and therefore improving the longevity of total joint replacements.

Wearing Out

Wearing of the implant is a problem that mainly affects total hip and knee replacements. Improvements in design, along with advances in bioengineering and materials technology, has substantially reduced the incidence of this problem and improved the life of the implant. The longevity of an implant depends on a number of factors, including the patient's weight, age, and activity level, but on average, current implants are expected to last, in the absence of complications, 10 to 20 years.

Metal Allergy

Allergy to the metals used in the construction of a total joint replacement is exceedingly rare. Most patients will already know about an allergy if one exists. Nevertheless, in occasional cases persistent pain and swelling may be due to this reaction. Allergy testing can then be carried out.

Pain

We have found that the majority of patients will progress through their surgery and rehabilitation without a hiccup. They will fall within the average time frames for recovery and progress through all the milestones within average limits. We would expect a hip or knee replacement patient to be walking independently or perhaps with one cane by 6 weeks. The patient should be pain-free, apart perhaps from some mild residual irritation at the site of the incision, and have a good functional range of motion. They will continue to improve for up to 1 year, as the tissues recover and the body gets used to the new joint. Always remember, everyone is different and people recover at different rates. Some may move a little faster and others may need a little extra time. Everyone's perception and tolerance of pain is different: what might be a minor irritation to one individual may cause severe limitation in another.

One of the hardest things to evaluate as an orthopedic surgeon is the patient who has persistent pain from a total joint replacement despite appearing to have a technically good result. The surgery and rehabilitation may have progressed smoothly, the joint looks excellent with regards to range of motion, healing, and lack of swelling, and the x-rays show no obvious problems. A situation like this is disappointing for both the patient and the surgeon as it is not the outcome expected by either. With appropriate investigations and management, most problems can be cleared up in time. Occasionally, despite our best efforts, the cause for the pain remains elusive. Your surgeon will generally ask for a second opinion to ensure that nothing has been missed. In these unusual cases, the patient is encouraged to remain active in the anticipation that the discomfort will generally settle. Pain management programs may be beneficial, which would include both natural therapies, such as acupuncture, medications, and nerve blocks.

Scar Tenderness
The surgical scar takes over 1 year to heal completely. You will know when it has healed, as it will turn from red to white. Some patients experience ongoing scar tenderness, which can be quite bothersome. Treatment with massage, ultrasound, and desensitization techniques generally allow this to settle. To reduce scarring, a zinc supplement and glucosamine sulphate may be beneficial.

Bursitis
Bursitis is a relatively common problem, particularly following total hip replacement. The pain occurs generally over the outside of the hip underneath the scar. It is quite tender to direct pressure, making it difficult to lie on that side. A similar problem can occur over the front of the knee.

Treatment is quite straightforward, involving modalities to reduce swelling, anti-inflammatory treatment, and occasionally injection of anaesthetic and cortisone. Acupuncture can be useful in bursitis.

Muscle Pain

Individuals undergoing a total joint replacement have often waited quite sometime for the procedure. During that period, their activity may have been severely curtailed by ongoing pain in the joint. The muscles can become deconditioned. When patients suddenly find themselves with a mobile, pain-free joint, they are keen to resume all their normal activities and hobbies. Unfortunately, many of the tissues, such as the muscles, don't recover with quite such enthusiasm. They will be sore and stiff for a number of months until they regain their strength and flexibility. Addition of a calcium/magnesium supplement, adequate hydration, massage, and contrast therapy are likely to be beneficial.

Altered Alignment

The new joint replacement will often alter the alignment of a limb. The body has been used to this alignment for many years and it may therefore take a number of months before the body, its ligaments and muscles, accommodate this new arrangement. This can be a source of discomfort. Massage and orthotic treatment may be effective, along with bromelain, devil's claw, and glucosamine complex supplements.

Pain from Other Joints

Arthritis can affect a number of joints at the same time. Although a patient might be acutely aware of one particular joint because it is so painful, once the pain has been relieved by a joint replacement, other joints may start to be bothersome. The pain from these other joints may be felt in the region of the new joint. This is particularly the case in arthritis of the hip, which can often cause pain in the knee. Pain from the back can also be referred to the hip or knee and may be aggravated by the strenuous efforts of rehabilitation and the newly acquired activity level.

FUTURE TREATMENT
OF ARTHRITIS

Research into the treatment of arthritis continues to progress at a fever-ish pace. With an aging population that is fitter and more active then ever before, the demand for better arthritis treatments is increasing. There arc several treatments that are largely experimental at this stage and gen-erally only available in a few specialised centers as part of a clinical trial. While these techniques appear promising and seem to offer tremendous advantages over many of the available techniques, their success and longevity remains to be proven.

Cartilage Transplantation

Until relatively recently, it was felt that the cells (chondrocytes) within the articular cartilage that covers the end of the bones at a joint were not capable of replication (dividing to form new cells). These cells are needed if articular cartilage is to be replaced or repaired, as they alone are capable of rebuilding the tissue that has been damaged. It does not appear that other cells are capable of doing this. Simply bringing blood supply to the area of damage as attempted with so called abrasion arthroplasty (a technique in which the exposed bone was burred away to create bleeding) seems to result only in unstable weak fibrous cartilage that is unable to withstand any significant force.

Isolated areas of cartilage damage with surface loss is one of the earliest changes seen in osteoarthritis. When these injuries occur as a result of trauma in younger individuals, they place them at risk of development of earlier arthritis. Full thickness defects larger than a few millimeters in diameter have been shown not to heal. This is primarily due to the absence of chondro-progenitor cells (cartilage stem cells) that have tremendous ability to replicate and create new cartilage matrix. Techniques to introduce these cartilage stem cells into damaged areas of cartilage have been developing since the 1980s. Studies have shown that the cartilage developed in this technique is very similar to articular cartilage. Appearance, microscopic evaluation, and mechanical testing have shown that this cartilage has a structure and properties similar to that of normal articular cartilage. Good to excellent results are seen in up to 85% percent of patients for up to 8 years. Most failures occur within the first 2 years.

Further research in this field is concentrating on the development of biodegradable scaffold within which the cartilage stem cells can be transplanted in order to improve the strength, characteristics, and structure of the newly formed cartilage. More complex techniques involve the creation of three-dimensional cartilage in the laboratory prior to implantation into the knee.

Mosaicplasty

Mosaicplasty is a more widely available treatment for cartilage defects than cartilage transplantation. Mosaicplasty involves the resurfacing of a damaged area of joint surface with good cartilage from another area not subject to loading during normal movement. This is similar to hair plug transplantation.

Experience has shown that the transplanted material survives well and is rapidly incorporated. Care must be taken to avoid taking the transplant cartilage from an area that may potentially interfere with the function of the joint. Initial use of the technique was in very small areas of cartilage loss, but as experience has been gained, areas between one and four centimeters are considered appropriate. Beyond this, technical difficulties and the availability of transplantable tissue cause problems.

When appropriate patients are selected, results are excellent. Good to excellent results are quoted in up to 92% of patients.

Tissue Engineering

Techniques in tissue engineering, in which the body's own reparative processes are enhanced and modified to promote or accelerate healing, is still very experimental. Growth factors have been identified and can conceivably be introduced to areas of damage to promote a healing response.

Genetic Engineering

A gene has been recently identified in mice that seems to influence the development of arthritis. One theory as to the initial change in arthritis is thought to be a thickening of the bony layer just beneath the surface of the joint. This gene may prevent arthritis by preventing the build up of crystals in this bony layer. A human version of this gene has been identified in an area known to be associated with joint disease. In the future, genetic modification or immunization may prevent or slow the development of arthritis.

Glossary

Absorption: The selective taking-in or abstraction of water or other materials from the alimentary canal (digestive tract) into the blood or lymphatic system.

Acupuncture: The process of inserting needles into specific points of meridians on the body to promote the increased flow of Qi or energy and promote healing.

Adenosine Triphoshate (ATP): A compound containing three phosphates that when broken down produces energy and enables muscles and organs to function.

Analgesics (painkillers): The first line in the medicinal treatment of arthritis.

Ankylosing Spondylitis: A type of inflammatory arthritis associated with the gene HLA-B27, most commonly presenting with back pain.

Antibody: A protein produced by the immune system that binds to an antigen to neutralize or destroy it.

Antigen: A substance recognized as foreign to the body inducing antibody formation against it.

Arthritis: Inflammation of a joint. Several different forms exist.

Arthralgia: Literally means pain in a joint. While arthritis does present with arthralgia, not all arthralgia is arthritis. Arthralgia is common in illness such as influenza.

Arthrodesis: A fusion of the joint such that no movement is allowed following the surgery.

Arthrography: Radiological technique in which dye is injected into a joint prior to the taking of x-rays.

Arthropathy: Damage or dysfunction within a joint.

Arthroplasty: Creation of a new joint. Most commonly refers to the replacement of a damaged joint (total joint replacement arthroplasty).

Arthroscopy: A minimally-invasive surgical technique used to evaluate and treat problems within certain joints. It is now the most commonly performed orthopedic procedure.

Articular: Relating to a joint.

Articular Cartilage: The smooth cartilage covering the end of a bone at a joint.

Anti-oxidant: A substance that neutralizes free radicals in the body. This aids the body in faster recover and promotes stronger, more healthy tissues.

Auto-immunity: An immune response produced by the body against one of its own cells or tissues.

Avascular Necrosis: A condition in which the blood supply to an area of bone is lost resulting in bone death and collapse.

Bioavailable: Easily absorbed and used by the body.

Biochemical Reactions: The chemical activities associated with life as exhibited in humans and other living organisms. These are the reactions that drive all bodily functions.

Biomechanics: The study of the way in which the body is constructed and moves.

Bone Bruising: A recent injury identified at the joint surface is that of a bone bruise. The injury was only made visible by the availability of MRI examination of the joint following trauma.

Bone Scan: This test measures 'bone cell activity'. It involves injection of a (non-harmful) radioactive marker into a vein in the hand, followed, 2 hours later, by a scan of the whole body or a specific area. Active areas show up as 'hot spots'.

Boron: Boron is a trace mineral that was only recently discovered as helpful to humans in the repair of bone and joints. It is found widely in fruits and vegetables.

Boswellia: Boswellia is a small tree native to India that has a gummy resin. This resin contains potent anti-inflammatory properties.

Bromelain: Bromelain contains enzymes naturally found in pineapple. Several beneficial results have been achieved by using these proteolytic enzymes as anti-inflammatory agents.

Bursa: One of the many protective sacks that occur throughout the body. The bursa is a slippery sack lined with the same tissue that lines a joint, synovial membrane. They provide cushioning and lubrication between structures.

Bursitis: Inflammation of a bursa (see *bursa*) causing pain and swelling.

Capsicum: Capsicum, found in the chili pepper, red pepper, or cayenne pepper, is one of the oldest spices now used therapeutically, usually in topical form, for its anti-inflammatory effects.

Carbohydrate: An organic compound in nature consisting of carbon, hydrogen, and oxygen that is used by the body as a potential fuel source. This includes starches, sugars, fiber, cellulose, and gums.

Cartilage: A complex composite connective tissue that covers the surfaces of bone (articular cartilage), providing strength and shock absorption to a joint. Other forms of cartilage exist throughout the body.

CAT Scan: CT or computer tomography uses x-rays from different angles to give a 3-dimensional image of the body.

Chiropractic Treatment: The gentle movement of joints and the surrounding musculature for therapeutic purposes.

Chondrocyte: A mature cartilage cell.

Chondroitin: A mixture of hydrolyzed GAGs (glycosaminoglycans) and sugars. It function is to inhibit the enzymes that break down collagen, and to provide building materials for cartilage.

Chondrogenic: Potential to promote cartilage growth or regeneration. Relating to cartilage.

Chondromalacia: Refers to deterioration in the quality of the articular cartilage that overlies the end of a bone at a joint.

Corticosteroids (hormones): A group of hormones synthesized in the adrenal glands. They have a multitude of effects, including control of the absorption and movement of fluids in the body, metabolism of glucose, and the control of inflammatory reactions in the body.

Cortisone (injection): A long acting form of the anti-inflammatory medicine used for injection into a joint.

Collagen: Long, chain-like, structural protein that provides strength to many tissues, including cartilage.

Collagenase: An enzyme that breaks down collagen.

Co-enxyme: A substance that must be present with an enzyme to allow that enzyme to function.

Contrast Treatment: Alternating application of heat and cold. Contrast baths are particularly effective at reducing tissue swelling.

Copper: Copper is an essential trace mineral that is part of several important enzyme reactions in the body. It is the third most abundant mineral in the human body.

COX: Acronym referring to cyclo-oxygenase enzymes that initiate inflammation through the production of different chemicals.

Cryotherapy: Treatment with cold or ice.

Curcumin: Curcumin or tumeric is a perennial herb native to Southern Asia and is grown extensively in the Caribbean. It is a member of the ginger family and has similar anti-inflammatory properties.

Cyclo-oxygenase: Essential enzymes involved in the production of prostaglandins and other chemicals that mediate inflammation.

Cytokines: Molecules released during inflammation that act to modulate the immune response by acting on numerous cell and tissue types. Include the interleukins (ILs) and tumour necrosis factor (TNF).

Debridement: Procedure refers to the evaluation of a joint with arthroscopy and the treatment of damaged areas within the joint. It can be considered a 'spring clean up' or 'lube, oil and filter'.

Degenerative Joint Disease (DJD): Synonymous with arthritis.

Devil's Claw: Devil's claw or Harpago phytum is a herbaceous plant native to South Africa. It possesses anti-inflammatory qualities and is used in the treatment of arthritis.

Diathermy: A physical modality of treatment providing deep heating to tissues.

Dimethyl sulfoxide (DMSO): DMSO is a by-product from the wood industry. Once in the body, it is converted into MSM and is used for the repair and health of cartilage.

DMARD: Disease-modifying anti-rheumatic drug. Any one of a number of medications used in inflammatory arthritis to modify the immune response.

Double-blind Study: A type of clinical trial in which neither the subjects nor the examiner know which product is being taken in order to reduce bias in results.

Dysplasia: Abnormal formation or development.

Enzyme: One group of proteins produced in cells that are capable of greatly accelerating chemical reactions in the body without being broken down or consumed themselves.

Eicosapentaenoic Acid (EPA): An omega-3 fatty acid that is also known as omega-6 and is primarily found in fresh water fish.

Essential fatty acids (EFAs): Fatty acids that the body cannot manufacture and therefore have to be obtained from diet (e.g., linoleic acid, arachidonic acid).

Extra-articular: Outside or surrounding a joint.

Fatty Acids: Dietary fat molecules needed for cell membranes, hormones. and other chemicals. Divided into essential and non-essential.

Fracture: A break in any bone.

Free Radical: A highly reactive molecule that is known to injure cell membranes, damage DNA, and contribute to aging and degenerative illnesses.

Free Radical Scavenger: A substance, like an anti-oxidant, that seeks out and destroys free radicals in the body.

Frozen Shoulder: Also called adhesive capsulitis, this condition causes the shoulder to become painful and stiff.

Glycosaminoglycans (GAGs): Chemical building blocks for cartilage that attract water to maintain cushioning and resilience.

Ginger: Ginger or Zingiber is a herb that originated in the Orient and quickly spread worldwide for its therapeutic use in digestion and inflammation.

Glucosamine Sulfate: A combination of glutamine and sulfate used in the manufacture of GAGs to increase the strength and structure of cartilage, maintain synovial fluid, and inhibit damaging enzymes.

Glucagon: A hormone secreted by the pancreas that promotes the mobilization of sugar or glucose from stores in the body.

Gout: A form of crystal arthritis caused by a deposition of uric acid crystals.

Hormone: A chemical substance formed in one part of the body and transported to a different area where it has a regulatory effect on different functions.

Hyaluronic Acid: Hyaluronic acid (hyaluronan) is the most important GAG in articular joint cartilage and joint fluid.

Hydrotherapy: Hydrotherapy is the external use of water-based modalities for treatment.

Hyperinsulinemia: An excess of insulin secretion resulting in low blood sugar levels or hypoglycemia. Chronic high secretion leads to *insulin resistance*.

Hypertrophic Arthritis: Arthritis in which the body produces extra bone or cartilage.

Immunoglobulin: Antibody protein molecules in which one end is used for the recognition of foreign material (antigens) and the other end activates an immune response.

Inflammation: A complex interaction of chemicals and cells forming a pathway that results in pain, swelling, stiffness, and tissue damage.

Inflammatory Arthritis: Arthritis in which there is an identifiable, immune-based, inflammatory response, which results both in arthritis and damage to other tissues.

Interferential: Physical therapy modality that involves the application of two "interfering" medium frequency alternating currents. Beneficial effects include pain relief, control of swelling, reduced muscle wasting, improved flexibility, and muscle strength.

Interleukins: Molecules in the *cytokine* group, released during inflammation and acting to modulate the immune response by acting on numerous cell and tissue types.

Intra-articular: Within a joint.

Insulin: A protein hormone formed and secreted by the pancreas in response to a rise in blood sugar level. It promotes lipid synthesis as it stores the sugar from the blood as fat.

Insulin Resistance: A condition in which the body is insensitive and even resistant against the effects of insulin. In most cases, the body responds by producing even more insulin.

In vitro: Existing outside of a living cell or body. Pertaining to an artificial or manufactured environment.

In vivo: Existing within a living cell or body, either animal or plant in nature.

Leukotrienes: Arachidonic acid metabolic products, which, along with *prostaglandins,* act to mediate the inflammatory response.

Magnetotherapy: The use of magnets as a physical therapy.

Massage Therapy: The technique of manual manipulation of the soft tissue of the body. It is used to increase circulation, decrease pain and spasticity, and promote healing.

Matrix: The molecular 'mesh' comprised of glycosaminoglycans (GAGs) that attracts water in cartilage.

Methylsulfonylmethane (MSM): A naturally occurring sulfur containing compound used as structural building material for cartilage.

Metalloproteases: Enzymes that break down cartilage matrix.

MRI: Magnetic resonance imaging uses changing magnetic fields to image the different structures in the body. Different tissues have different 'resonance' properties, and these properties change if the tissue is inflamed or altered by disease.

Mosaicplasty: Involves the resurfacing of a damaged area of joint surface with good cartilage from another area that is not subject to loading during normal movement.

Myalgia: Pain in the muscles. Often associated with unaccustomed exercise or, as with arthralgia, associated with influenza.

Naturopathy: Medical practice using natural substances and treatments, such as diet, herbs, homeopathic remedies, and acupuncture, to stimulate the body's innate healing response and produce therapeutic effects.

Obesity: An excessive accumulation of fat in the body, mainly deposited in the subcutaneous tissues. It is generally considered 30% above normal body weight.

NSAID (Non-steroidal anti-inflammatory drug): Medication that includes ASA with a specific effect at controlling inflammation through inhibition of the prostaglandin pathway.

Occupational Therapy: Plays a pivotal role in the treatment and management of the arthritis patient. Patient education, particularly with reference to daily activity, is most valuable. Activity modification involves the adaptation of techniques, such as pacing and postural retraining, to minimize discomfort and maximize function. Design and manufacture of splints and aids.

Orthopedics: The division of surgery that deals with ailments of the locomotor system. Includes joints, muscles, ligaments, and tendons from the toes to the skull.

Orthotics: Inserts within footwear designed to aid the foot during walking and to improve biomechanics.

Osteoarthritis: Chronic arthritis or inflammation of a joint that is degenerative in nature. It is usually, but not always, associated with aging and obesity, and is not accompanied by involvement of remote tissues or organs (cf. *inflammatory arthritis).*

Osteoporosis: Loss of bone mass.

Osteotomy: Refers to the realignment of a bone above or below a joint in order to change the forces across the joint. Generally, the procedure is carried out to unload a damaged area of the joint.

Phospholipases: A group of enzymes that degrade the structural phospholipid layer that surrounds cells.

Physiotherapy: Incorporates education of the patient about an injury or disease process, discussion of their expectations, guidance and precautions with regards to activity. In addition, it incorporates passive and active stretching, strengthening, mobilization, posture and balance, as well as many physical modalities.

Placebo: An inactive substance used as a comparison in clinical tests.

Polyarticular: Involving a number of joints.

Prostaglandins: Arachidonic acid metabolic products, which, along with *leukotrienes,* act to mediate the inflammatory response.

Protein: A class of organic nitrogen-based compounds, essential structural components of all cells and the basis of the majority of active molecules in the body.

Protein Kinase: A generic term for an enzyme that phosphorylates (adds a phosphate to) protein.

Proteinase: Enzyme that breaks down protein.

Proteoglygans: A component of the extra cellular matrix or 'ground substance' of cartilage.

Pseudogout: An inflammatory arthritis of the joints caused by crystals of calcium pyrophosphate. It is also known as calcium pyrophosphate deposition disease (CPDD).

Psoriatic Arthritis: A type of inflammatory arthritis associated with the skin condition psoriasis.

Rheumatoid Arthritis: Rheumatoid arthritis is one of a number of inflammatory diseases that diffusely affect tissues and joints throughout the body.

Rheumatology: Medical specialty concerned with inflammatory diseases of joints and other tissues.

Sacroiliitis: Inflammation of the sacroiliac joints at the back of the pelvis.

S-Adenosylmethionine (SAM-e): Formed from the amino acid methionine and ATP, it increases proteoglycan production.

Saturated Fats: A fatty acid that has every possible bond filled with hydrogen atoms and is therefore less reactive. They tend to be solid at room temperature and generally are from an animal origin.

Shortwave Diathermy: Involves passage of a high frequency current with no nerve stimulation. The rapid vibration induces deep heat in the tissues.

Spondyloarthritis: Osteoarthritis of the spine.

Subchondral: Refers to the bone layer just beneath the cartilage in a joint.

Substance P: A neuroactive peptide or chemical messenger that is released from pain fibers.

Superoxide Dismutase: An enzyme produced in the body to scavenge free radicals and therefore decrease oxidation and inflammation.

Synovium: The tissue that lines every synovial joint, producing *synovial fluid*.

Synovial fluid: The viscous lubricating fluid within a joint.

Synovectomy: Removal of the synovial lining from a joint.

Tendonitis: Inflammation of a tendon.

Tenosynovitis: Inflammation of the sheath that surrounds a tendon.

Tumeric: Tumeric or curcumin is a perennial herb native to Southern Asia and is grown extensively in the Caribbean. It is a member of the ginger family and has similar anti-inflammatory properties.

Vitamin C: Also known as ascorbic acid, vitamin C is a water-soluble vitamin with anti-oxidant properties. Vitamin C also acts as a *co-enzyme* in several reactions in the body.

Vitamin E: Also known as tocopherol, vitamin E is a fat-soluble vitamin with anti-oxidant properties.

Ultrasound: Mechanical energy in the form of high frequency vibration, transmitted to tissues as a form of physical therapy.

Willow: Willow or salix is a well-known herb, also known as aspirin.

Yoga: The physical practice that uses strengthening and stretching to bring balance and healing to all aspects of the body, the emotional, mental, and physical.

Zinc: A mineral present in every cell in the body and a component in over 200 *enzyme* reactions.

References

Adams, M.E. et al. The role of viscosupplementation with hylan G-F 20 (Synvisc) in the treatment of osteoarthritis of the knee. *Osteoarthritis Cartilage*, 1995; Dec 3(4): 213-25.

Altman, R.D. Effects of a ginger extract on knee pain in patients with osteoarthritis. *Arthritis and Rheumatism*, 2001 (Nov);44(11):2531-538.

Altman, R.D. Efficacy and safety of Zinaxin in patients with osteoarthritis, a multi-centre Phase-III, placebo-controlled, double-blind, randomized, two–armed, five month, cross over study. *Arthritis and Rheumatism*, 2001:44(11):2531-539.

Ammon, H.P., Safayhi, H., Mack, T., Sabieraj, J. Mechanisms of antinflammatory action of curcumin and boswellic acid. *J. Ethnopharmacol* (Ireland), 1993; 38/2-3:113-19.

Arora, R., et al. Anti-inflammatory studies on curcuma longa (turmeric). *Indian J Med Res.*, 1971;59:1289-95.

Baici, A., et al., Analysis of GAG's in human serum after oral administration of chondroitin sulfate. *Rheumatol In*, 1992;12:81-88.

Brady, L.R. ,Tyler V.E., and Robbers, J.E. *Pharmacognosy*. 8th ed. Philadelphia: Lea and Febiger, 1981: 480.

Bucsi, L. and Poor, G. Efficacy and tolerability of oral chondroitin sulfate as a symptomatic slow-acting drug for osteoarthritis (SYSADOA) in the treatment of knee osteoarthritis. *Osteoarthritis Cartilage*, 1998;6 (Suppl A):31-36.

Burton, G.W. and Traber, M.G. Vitamin E: Anti-oxidant activity, biokinetics and bioavailability. *Annu Rev Nutr*, 1992;10:357-82.

Caperton, E.M. et al. Antibiotic therapy of chronic inflammatory arthritis archives. *Internal Medicine*, 1990;150:1677-682.

Caruso, I. and Peitrogrande, V. Italian double-blind multicenter study comparing S-adenosylmethionine, naproxen, and placebo in the treatment of degenerative joint disease. *Am J Med*, 1987;83(suppl 5A):66-71.

Chan, M.M. Inhibition of tumor necrosis factor by curcumin, a phytochemical. *Biochemical Pharmacology,* 1995;49(11):1551-556.

Cofield, R. H., Chang, W., and Spearling, J.W. *Complications of shoulder arthroplasty in disorders of the shoulder.* Philadelphia, PA: Lippincott, Williams and Wilkins, 1999.

Conte, A. et al. Biochemical and pharmakinetic aspects of oral treatment with chondroitin sulfate. *Arzneim Forsch,* 1995 (45):918-25.

Cook, S.D. et al. Improved cartilage repair with low intensity ultrasound. *CORR,* 2001: 391(S), S231-43.

Deal, C.L. and Moskowitz, R.W. Effect of glucosamine sulfate on chondrocytes in vitro. *Rheum Dis Clin North Am,* 1999; 25:3791.

Deal, C.L. et al. Treatment of arthritis with topical capsaicin: A double blind trial. *Clin Ther,* 1991;13:383-95.

del Puenta, Scarpa and Digirolamo, C. et al. Interplay between environmental factors, articular involvement and HLA-B27 in patients with psoriatic arthritis. *Ann Rheum Dis,* 1992; 51:78.

Deodhar, S.D., Sethi, R., Srimal, R.C. Preliminary studies on antirheumatic activity of curcumin (di-feruloyl methane). *Indian J Med Res,* 1980;71:632-34.

di Padova, C. S-adenosylmethionine in the treatment of osteoarthritis: Review of the clinical studies. *Am J Med,* 1987: (Suppl 5A):60-65.

Etzel, R. Special extracts of Boswellia serrata in the treatment of rheumatoid arthritis. *Phytomedicine,* 1996;3 (1):67-70.

ESCOP Monographs, Fascicule 2, Harpagophytum radix. 1996:1.

ESCOP Monographs, Fascicule 2, Harpagophytum radix. 1996:4.

ESCOP: Salicis Cortex/Willow Bark. In: ESCOP Monograph Fascicule 4. Exeter: ESCOP; 1997:58.

Ezza, J., Hadhazy, V., Birch, S., Lao, L., Kaplan, G., Hochberg, M., Berman, B. Acupuncture for osteoarthritis of the knee: a systematic review. *Arthritis Rheum,* 2001 (Apr);44(4):819-25.

Feibel, A. and Fast, A. Deep heating of joints – a reconsideration. *Archives Phys Med Rehabil,* 1978;59(8): 383.

Finley, E.B. and Cerklewski, F.L. Influence of ascorbic acid and copper in young adults. *Am J Clin Nutr,* 47; 1988:96-101.

Fox, R.B. and Fox, W.K. DMSO prevents hydroxyl radical-mediated depolymerization of hyaluronic acid. *Ann NY Acad Sci,* 1983;411:14-18.

Frondoza, C. et al. TNF expression of synoviocyte cultures is inhibited by hydroxy-alkoxy-phenyl compounds from ginger, John Hopkins University, Presented at *International Cartilage Repair Society Congress,* Sweden 2000.

Gabriel, S.E. and Conn, D.L. Rifamycin therapy in rheumatoid arthritis. *J Rheumatol,* 1990;17:160-66.

Garfinkel M.S., Schumacher H.R. Jr., Husain A., Levy, M., Reshetar, R.A. Evaluation of a yoga regimen for treatment of osteoarthritis of the hands. *J Rheumatol,* 1994 (Dec); 21(12): 2341-343.

Garfinkel, M. and Schumacher H.R. Jr. Yoga. *Rheum Dis Clin North Am,* 2000 (Feb); 26(1): 125-32.

Goldman, R.T., Scuderi, G.R., Kelly, M.A. Arthroscopic treatment of the degenerative knee in older athletes. *Clin Sports Med,* 1997;16:51-68.

Goto, M. et al. Intraarticular injection of hyaluronate improves joint pain and synovial fluid PGE-2 levels in rheumatoid arthritis. *Clin Exp Rheumatol,* 2001 (Jul-Aug);19(4):377-83.

Grahame, R. and Robinson, B. Devils' Claw (Harpagophytum procumbens): pharmacological and clinical studies. *Ann Rheum Dis,* 1981;40:632.

Hangody, L. et al. Mosiacplasty for the treatment of articular defects of the knee and ankle. *Clinical Orthopedics and Related Research,* 2001 (Oct);391-S: S328-336.

Harmand, M.F. et al. Effects of S-adenosylmethionine on human articular chondrocyte differentiation: An in vitro study. *Am J Med,* 83(Suppl 5A) 1987: 48-54.

Haslam, R. A comparison of acupuncture with advice and exercises on the random symptomatic treatment of osteoarthritis of the hip – a randomised controlled trial. *Acupunct Med,* 2001 (Jun);19(1):19-26.

Hungerford, D.S. Treating Osteoarthritis with chondroprotective agents. *Orthop Special Ed,* 1998;4910:39-42.

Inman, R.D. Antigens, the gastrointestinal tract and arthritis. *Rheum Dis Clin,* 1991;17:309-320.

Jacob, S.W. and Herschler, R. DMSO after twenty years. *Ann NY Acad Sci,* 1983:411, xiii-xvii.

Johnson, A.H. and Kingsley, D.M. Role of the mouse ANK gene in control of tissue calcification and arthritis. *Science,* 2000;289:265-70.

Kolb, K.H., Jaenicke, Kramer, M. et al. Absorption, distribution and elimination of labeled DMSO in man and animals. *Ann NY Acad Sci,* 1967;141:85-95.

Kremer, J.M., Jubiz, W., Michalek, A. et al. Fish-oil acid supplementation in active rheumatoid arthritis. A double-blinded, controlled, cross-over study. *Ann Intern Med,* 1987;106:497-503.

Kulkarni, R.R. et al. Treatment of osteoarthritis with a herbomineral formulation: A double-blind, placebo-controlled, cross-over study. *J Ethnopharmacol,* 1991 (May-Jun);33:91-95.

Lockie, L.M. and Norcross, B. A clinical study of the effects of DMSO in 103 patients with acute and chronic musculoskeletal injuries and inflammation. *Ann NY Acad Sci,* 1967;141:599-602.

Locock, R.A. Capsicum, *Canadian Parmaceutical Journal,* 1985;118:517-19.

Lopez, D. Double-blind clinical evaluation of the relative efficacy of ibuprofen and glucosamine sulphate in the management of osteoarthritis of the knee in out-patients. *Curr Med Res Opin,* 1982; 8(3):145-49.

Lunec, J. and Blake, D.R. The determinations of dehydroascorbic acid and ascorbic acid in the serum and synovial fluid of patients with rheumatoid arthritis. *Free Radic Res Comm,* 1985;1:31-39.

Mantzioris, E. et al., Dietary substitution with alpha-linolenic acid rich vegetable oil increases eicosapentaenoic acid concentrations in tissues. *Am J Clin Nutr,* 1994;59: 1304-309.

Matsui, N. et al., Arthroscopic versus open synovectomy in the rheumatoid knee. *Internat Orthop,* 1989;13:17-20.

Matsumoto, J. Clinical trials of DMSO in rheumatoid arthritic patients in Japan. *Ann NY Acad Sci,* 1967;141:560-68.

Mattingly, P.C. and Mowat, A.G. Zinc sulfate in rheumatoid arthritis. *Annals of the Rheumatic Diseases,* 1982;41:456-57.

McCaleb, Leung, A.Y., Foster, S. *Encyclopedia of Common Natural Ingredients Used in Foods, Drugs and Cosmetics.* 2nd ed. New York, NY: John Wiley and Sons, 1996:649.

McCleane, G. The analgesic efficacy of topical capsaicin is enhanced by glyceryl trinitrate in painful osteoarthritis. *Eur J Pain,* 2000;4(4):355-60.

Muller-Fassbender, H. Double-blind clinical trial of S-adenosylmethionine versus ibuprofen in the treatment of Osteoarthritis. *Am J Med,* 1987;83 (suppl 5A):81-83.

Murray, M.T. *The Healing Power of Herbs.* Rocklin, CA: Prima Publishing, 1992:246.

Murray, M. *Encyclopedia of Natural Medicine.* 2nd ed. Rocklin, CA: Prima Publishing, 1998:783.

Nielsen, F.H. et al. Effects of dietary boron on mineral, estrogen and testosterone in post-menopausal women. *Environ Health Perspect,* 1987:1:394-97.

Newnham, R.E. Essentiality of boron for healthy bones and joints. *Environ Health Perspect,* 1994:102 (suppl 7):83-85.

Ogilvie-Harris, D.J. and Basinski, A. Arthroscopic synovectomy of the knee for rheumatoid arthritis. *Arthroscopy,* 1991;7:91-97.

Palmbald, J., Hofsstrom, I., Ringetz, B. Antirheumatic effects of fasting. *Rheum Dis Clin,* 1991;17:351-62.

Parcell, S. Sulfur in human nutrition and applications in medicine. *Alternative Medical Review,* 2002 (Feb);7(1):22-44.

Peterson, L. et al. Autologous chondrocyte transplantation. *American Journal of Sports Medicine,* 2002; 30(1):2-12.

Petrella, R.J., DiSilvestro, M.D., Hildebrand, C. Effects of hyaluronate sodium on pain and physical functioning in osteoarthritis of the knee. *Arch Intern Med,* 2002 (Feb 11);162(3):292-98.

Pinget, M. and Lecomte, A. The effects of harpagophytum capsules (arkocaps) in degenerative rheumatology. *Medicine Actuelle,* 1985;12:65-67.

Piperno, M., Reboul, P., Le Graverand, M.P., Pershard, M.J., Annefeld, M., Richard, M., Vignon, E. Glucosmaine sulfate modulates dysregulated activites of human osteoarthritic chondrocyes in vitro. *Osteoarthritis and Cartilage,* 2000 (May); 8(3):207-12.

Prins, A.P., Lipman, J.M., McDevitt, C.A., Sokoloff, L. Effects of purified growth factors on rabbit chondrocytes in monolayer cultures. *Arthr Rheum,* 1982;25:1228-232.

Puett, D.W., and Griffin, M.R. Published trials of nonmedical and noninvasive therapies for hip and knee osteoarthritis. *Ann Intern Med,* 1994;121(2):133-40.

Reginster, J.Y., Deroisy, R., Rovati, L.C., Lee, R.L., Lejeune, E., Bruyere, O., Giacovelli, G., Henrotin, Y., Dacre, J.E., Gossett, C. Long term effects of glucosamine sulfate on osteoarthritis progression: a randomized, placebo-controlled clinical trial. *Lancet,* 2001 (Jan 27); 357 (9252):247-8:11214122.

Richmond, V.L. Incorporation of methylsulfonylmethane sulfate into guinea pig serum protein. *Life Science,* 1986;39:263-68.

Rizzo, R., Grandolfo, Godeas C. et al. Calcium, sulfur and zinc distribution in normal and arthritic equine cartilage. *Exp Zool,* 1995;273:82-86.

Robbins, W. Clinical applications of capsaicinoids. *Clin J Pain,* 2000 (June);16(2 suppl.):S86-89.

Ronca, F. et al. Anti-inflammatory activity of chondroitin sulfate. *Osteoarthritis Cartilage,* 1998;6(Suppl A):14-21.

Ronca, F. et al. Anti-inflammatory activity of chondroitin sulfate. *Osteoarthritis Cartilage,* 1998;6 (Suppl A):14-21.

Sansone, P. and Schmitt, L. Providing tender touch massage to elderly nursing home residents: a demonstration project. *Geriatr Nurs,* 2000 (Nov-Dec);21(6):303-08.

Schwartz, E.R. The modulation of osteoarthritic development by vitamins C and E. *J Vit Nutr Res,* 1984; (Suppl 26):141-46.

Setnikar, I. and Rovati, L.C. Absorption, distribution, metabolism and excretion of glucosamine sulfate. *Arzneimittelforschung,* 2001 (Sept);51(9):699-725.

Sperling, R.I., Weinblatt, M., Robin, J. et al. Effects of dietary supplementation with marine fish oil on leukocyte lipid mediator generation and function in rheumatoid arthritis. *Arthritis Rheum,* 1987;30:988-97.

Srivastave, K.C. and Mustafa, T. Ginger (zingiber officinale) rheumatism and musculoskeletal disorders. *Medical Hypothesis,* 1992;39:342-48.

Tanabe, M., Chen, Y-D., Saito, K-I., Kano, Y. Cholesterol biosynthesis inhibitory component from Zingiber officinale roscoe. *Chemical and Pharmaceutical Bulletin,* 1993;41(4):710-13.

Tanger, R. Ginger and atractylodes as an anti-inflammatory. *Herbalgram,* 1993;29:19.

Tapadinhas, M.J., Rivera, L.C., Bignamin, A.A. Oral glucosamine sulfate in management of arthrosis: report on multicentre open investigation in Portugal. *Pharmatherapeutica,* 1982;3(3):157-68.

Thie, N.M., Prasad, N.G., Major, P.W. Evaluation of glucosamine sulfate compared to ibuprofen for treatment of temporomandibular joint osteoarthritis: A randomized double blind controlled 3 month clinical trial. *Journal of Rheum,* 2001 (Jan);28(6):1347-355.

Tilwe, G.H., Beria, S., Turakhia, N.H., Daftary, G.V., Schiess, W. Efficacy and tolerability of oral enzymes therapy as compared to diclofenac in active osteoarthritis of knee joint: An open randomized controlled clinical trial. *J Assoc Physicians India,* 2001 (June);49:617-21.

Towheed, T.E. et al. Glucosamine therapy for treating arthritis from the community. Health and Epidemiology, Queen's University, Kingston, Ontario. *Cochrane Database Syst Rev.*

Travers, R.L., Rennie, G.C., Newnham, R.E. Boron and arthritis: The results of a double blind pilot study. *J Nutr Med,* 1990;1:27-32.

Tyler, V. *Herbs of Choice. The Therapeutic Use of Phytochemicinals.* Binghampton, NY: Pharmaceutical Products Press; 1994:209.

Under, A., Trang, L., Venizelos, N., Palmblad, J. Neutrophil function and clinical performance after total fasting in patients with rheumatoid arthritis. *Ann Rheum Dis,* 1983:42:45-51.

Verma, S., Singh, J., Khamesra, R., Bordia, A. Effect of ginger on platelet aggregation in man. *Indian J Med Res,* 1993;98:240-42.

Vetter, G. Double-blind comparative clinical trial with S-adenosylme-thionine versus indomethacin in the treatment of osteoarthritis. *Am J Med,* 1987;83 (suppl 5A):78-80.

Wai, E.K. et al. Arthroscopic debridement of the knee for osteoarthritis in patients fifty years of age or older. *JBJS,* 2002 (Jan);84-A(1):17-22.

Walker, W.R. and Keats, D.M. An investigation on the therapeutic value of the "copper bracelet": Dermal assimilation of copper in arthrits/rheumatoid conditions. *Agents Actions,* 1976;6454-459.

Wawrzynska-Pagowska, J. and Brzczinska, B. A. Trial of ampicillin in the treatment of rheumatoid arthritis results of long-term observations. *Rheumatologia,* 1994; 22:1-10.